"This contribution is the single most unequivocal academic reminder that the medicine is living art. I've never read a text that testifies so strongly to the metaphor and poetry of what we can do."

Russell Brown LAc, author of *Maya Angelou's Meditation 1814*

"Dr. Farrell's exploration of the 8 EVs is nuanced with practical, personal and deeply insightful candor. She demystifies the 8 EVs and preserves their profound intent to support the spiritual journey."

Luke Adler LAc, author of *Born to Heal*

PSYCHO-EMOTIONAL PAIN and the
EIGHT EXTRAORDINARY VESSELS

of related interest

Eight Extraordinary Channels – Qi Jing Ba Mai
A Handbook for Clinical Practice and Nei Dan Inner Meditation
Dr David Twicken DOM, LAc
ISBN 978 1 84819 148 8
eISBN 978 0 85701 137 4

Acupuncture and Chinese Medicine
Roots of Modern Practice
Charles Buck
ISBN 978 1 84819 159 4
eISBN 978 0 85701 133 6

Intuitive Acupuncture
John Hamwee
ISBN 978 1 84819 273 7
eISBN 978 0 85701 220 3

The Luo Collaterals
A Handbook for Clinical Practice and Treating Emotions
and the Shen and The Six Healing Sounds
Dr David Twicken DOM, LAc
ISBN 978 1 84819 230 0
eISBN 978 0 85701 219 7

The Active Points Test
A Clinical Test for Identifying and Selecting Effective
Points for Acupuncture and Related Therapies
Stefano Marcelli
ISBN 978 1 84819 233 1
eISBN 978 0 85701 207 4

PSYCHO-EMOTIONAL PAIN
and the
EIGHT EXTRAORDINARY VESSELS

YVONNE R. FARRELL

Foreword by David Chan
Illustrations by DevDiem Studios

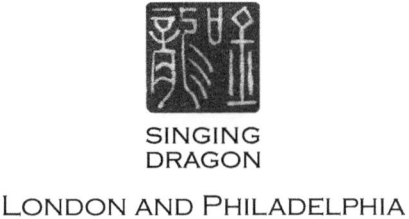

SINGING
DRAGON

LONDON AND PHILADELPHIA

First published in 2016
by Singing Dragon
an imprint of Jessica Kingsley Publishers
73 Collier Street
London N1 9BE, UK
and
400 Market Street, Suite 400
Philadelphia, PA 19106, USA

www.singingdragon.com

Library of Congress Cataloging in Publication Data
Names: Farrell, Yvonne R., author.
Title: Psycho-emotional pain and the eight extraordinary vessels / Yvonne R.
    Farrell ; foreword by David Chan.
Description: London ; Philadelphia : Singing Dragon, 2016. | Includes
    bibliographical references and index.
Identifiers: LCCN 2016001391 | ISBN 9781848192928 (alk. paper)
Subjects: | MESH: Acupuncture Points | Medicine, Chinese Traditional |
    Stress, Psychological--therapy
Classification: LCC RM184 | NLM WB 369.5.M5 | DDC 615.8/92-
    -dc23 LC record available at http://lccn.loc.gov/2016001391

British Library Cataloguing in Publication Data
A CIP catalogue record for this book is available from the British Library

ISBN 978 1 84819 292 8
eISBN 978 0 85701 239 5

Printed and bound in Great Britain

For Nate,
my favorite teacher.
I have learned more from you
about the nature of suffering than could
have been gleaned from a thousand patients.
You have taught me much about the necessity
of hope and the comfort found in a brief moment
of grace or an unexpected fit of the giggles.
I love you more than you can imagine.
Mom

DISCLAIMER

The information in this book is based on the author's knowledge and personal experience. This information is presented for educational purposes only. It is meant to aid the reader in developing a deeper understanding of Chinese Medicine. The diagnosis and point prescriptions are to be used at the reader's own discretion and liability. The author is not responsible in any manner for any injury that might occur as a result of following the recommendations in this book.

CONTENTS

FOREWORD

It is especially gratifying to see a student become a practitioner, teacher and then a master in her own right. Such is the pathway that I have witnessed in Yvonne Farrell's growth and transformation. When life steers you to the esoteric it's nice to have somebody to talk with and exchange ideas. I am grateful to have shared in that collaborative process. In this she has excelled every step of the way.

This book lays down a framework and then dives into the core issues. Destiny, purpose, the meaning of life and the nature of suffering are not to be taken lightly. The Daoists and Buddhists say that suffering occurs when we don't understand our pain. If we can see cause and effect then we can make conscious choices. There are those who think that their health is somehow disconnected from their lifestyles. This book is not for them unless they can open their minds to another perspective.

We tend to avoid consciousness of pain. We try to make it go away before we have even perceived its nature, intensity, movement, etc. Western medicine is based upon science, with spirituality being a topic that is either ignored or refuted and very seldom embraced. So pharmaceuticals are chemistry's answer to symptoms of various illnesses. There is no question that this is useful and necessary in many instances. But the use of more natural techniques with less or no side effects could be explored first if the situation hasn't grown to dire proportions. Listening to the body's reactions is a key component of this book. How do we work to understand and change the situation and not just suppress it? As the number of pharmaceuticals we ingest increases, so do the side effects and we lose sight of the original health picture and become mired in complications.

Classical Chinese Medicine is rich with thousands of years of evolution. It is still evolving. Daoists and Buddhists honor individual expression of these timeless precepts. Yvonne's interpretation and cultivation of the medicine is reflected in her clinical experience and expertise. Embodying the principles in her practice, her classes and her writings, she has taken her place in this distinguished lineage.

She and I are followers of Jeffrey Yuen and the Jade Purity School of Daoism. Like the master she learned from, she is modeling methods of treatment, not giving you specific treatments but rather showing you her thought process and analysis. In this book she is showing you a way to treat, a mindset rather than a point prescription. Jeffrey has taught her well.

David Chan OMD, LAc

ACKNOWLEDGMENTS

Although writing a book is a solitary endeavor, no one really ever writes a book alone. The writer's knowledge, experience and wisdom are derived from their relationships. If I were to thank everyone who contributed to this book by being part of my experiences this would be longer than the book itself. So even if you are not mentioned here, please know that I am grateful for you in my life.

Gratitude first for my teachers, especially Jeffrey Yuen and David Chan. Your teachings inspired me and I am forever changed by your wisdom, compassion and generosity.

Many thanks to the students who opened their hearts and minds to me. You have taken what I have taught, embodied it and used it to ease the suffering of others. I feel blessed.

Thank you to Claire Wilson and her team at Singing Dragon. As a first-time author I had no idea what I was getting into but I knew you wanted me to have a book that would make me proud. Thank you so much for your support and hard work.

To those who read the manuscript and gave feedback and encouragement, thank you.

A special thanks to Nate and his compadres at DevDiem Studios, Primo, Cody and Spencer for illustrations that are educational and still have plenty of attitude.

Thank you, thank you, thank you Russell Brown. This book would not have happened without your enthusiastic nudging and honesty. It was sometimes overwhelming but always enlivening to see myself through your eyes. The heart in this book came at your urging.

Last but by no means least, I would like to thank Trace Albrecht and Laura Erlich. Your support over the last decade has given me the ability to stretch myself while knowing that I was not alone. You have been the best cheerleaders a girl could ask for.

PREFACE

Chinese Medicine (CM) has an "inner tradition" which recognizes that medicine can be used as a tool to aid in spiritual development. Physical, emotional and mental illness is directly correlated to the degree in which an individual is capable of living his/her destiny. There is evidence of this in both the classic literature of CM and the current literature of acupuncture, metaphysics and psychological disciplines.

The modern day works of people like Jeffrey Yuen, Heiner Freuhauf, Mikio Sankey, Lonny Jarrett, Caroline Myss and Deepak Chopra all have some basis in the philosophy that the cultivation of consciousness is a vital part of the pursuit of health, meaning and purpose in life.

It became apparent to me early in my learning that when treated by skilled practitioners with appropriate Traditional Chinese Medicine (TCM) principles, a significant number of patients did not get better or had some relief from symptoms but those symptoms eventually returned. When I was doing my internship at school we had many patients who came weekly for treatment. They loved acupuncture and felt that the acupuncture really helped them and yet when you looked at their chief complaints you could easily see that their original issues were still there. I think that is because the focus was on the physical symptoms and did not acknowledge that all illness is an illness of the soul or that physical pain or suffering has its root in a psycho-spiritual or psycho-emotional disharmony.

Does this mean that when someone stubs their toe causing pain they are out of alignment in a spiritual sense? In a word, yes. However, it is probably not necessary to treat that toe pain as a spiritual imbalance. Treating the pain is what the patient needs at the time. If that patient is continually stubbing their toes or causing themselves pain or injury then surely it must be the practitioner's duty to help the patient ascertain why they are so clearly unaware of their surroundings. "What is stopping you from being fully present in your body?" This is a spiritual issue, an issue of consciousness, and continuing to treat the physical pain without addressing the imbalance of spirit does not fully serve the patient.

In most of the schools in the US, students learn the primary channel system as the main acupuncture system in CM. This system fits very well with the zangfu or organ theory that is used in herbal medicine. They complement each other well. But the primary channels are not the only channels available to acupuncturists. Rather they are a sort of middle of the road system that gives the student a useful and comprehensive system for approaching illness. This system is excellent for acute physical symptoms or for supporting the deficiencies of the body. It can also be helpful in addressing acute emotional distress. I am by no means suggesting that the primary channels be dismissed as ineffective. Their effect is often profound and it can help patients to survive a crisis until they are ready to deal with the underlying spiritual imbalance. The system of the primary channels can bring about a balance in the physical body; it is not in my experience comprehensive enough to deal with existential crises. The search for self is a deeper matter.

I began to search for ways to address that missing piece. The first glimpse of hope came from my teacher, mentor and friend David Chan OMD. David introduced me to the Secondary Vessels and Taoist theory. He also introduced me to Taoist monk Jeffrey Yuen whose classes inspired me to integrate what I already knew about spirit into my assessment and treatment of my patients by using the Secondary Vessels, especially the Eight Extraordinary Vessels.

The theories of the Secondary Vessels are minimally taught in the US schools of TCM. They are used even less in the schools. This may be in part because of the limitation of time. Most of the time spent in school focuses on the primary channels. Chinese Medical Theory is taught using the primary channels, the organs they are associated with and the herbal theories that apply to the organ functions. That is a lot to learn in just a few short years.

Acupuncture has a much greater scope than just the primary channels. The channel system extends from wei qi down into yuan qi and expresses itself at these differing levels through additional sub-systems that are sometimes known as these Secondary Vessels.

They are as follows:

- the Tendino-muscular Meridians (TMMs)

- the luo-collaterals

- the Divergent Meridians

- the Eight Extraordinary Vessels (8 EV).

The first three are considered extensions of, or related to, the primary meridians. The last system of vessels is actually a precursor to the primary meridians and therefore might be thought of as the vessels that contain the seed of destiny planted by the will of Heaven at the moment of conception. To fulfill our destiny this seed has to be nourished in the course of our lives.

THE EIGHT EXTRAORDINARY VESSELS (8 EV)

As the precursors for the primary meridians, the 8 EV are considered prenatal vessels. In TCM, these vessels are frequently used to treat constitutional issues. In particular, it is fairly common to see these vessels used in combination with the primary meridians in the treatment of infertility, neurological disorders and psycho-emotional conditions. They are typically not fully recognized and used as an autonomous system in TCM.

If we broaden our view of these vessels we can see their intimate relationship to the function of the kidneys in TCM. The kidneys, being the source of yuan qi in the primary channel system, can also be associated with the truest aspect of who we are. Therefore these vessels connect us to our authentic self.

It is through these vessels that the development of personality happens. Carl Jung and Caroline Myss both speak of this development in terms of archetypes. At different times in our lives we are living mythic roles. In childhood we may be living through the archetype of the wounded child or perhaps we are living the myth of the magical child. As a young adult, a woman might live through the archetype of the prostitute or the victim. This does not mean she becomes a prostitute. Rather it means she has come to a stage in her life when she must negotiate some of the feelings and energies that are typical in those who live a life of prostitution. She must find her worth. In later adulthood she might live out one of archetypes of the mother or crone. These archetypes can be very helpful in terms of our development of consciousness but we can also get "stuck" in them. When patients get stuck in the archetypes, pathology is most often apparent in one or more of the 8 EV.

What follows in this book is an exploration of the 8 EV from the point of view of suffering. Little time will be spent on the physiological conditions that are associated with these vessels. That information can be found in any number of good texts. The focus will be on how the 8 EV represent the unfolding of jing and how that is expressed in the pursuit of one's destiny. This is an exploration of the nature of suffering that is created by a resistance to life's experiences.

This book has two parts. Part 1 lays down a framework for the nature of suffering and the body's self-preservation mechanisms. It explores how the psyche communicates through the body by creating physical discomfort that is supposed to initiate the need for change. It investigates each of the 8 EV and their pathways, points and what part each vessel plays in how jing unfolds. Part 2 contains suggestions on how to create an 8 EV treatment and case studies that come directly from my practice. Although this section includes diagnostic information and point prescriptions, it is not a clinical manual. This is not about protocols for treating conditions. It is about an approach to seeing your patients that includes their resistance to change, the nature of their suffering and a way to create a therapeutic environment that allows for the possibility of change.

I hope it sheds a little light on these beautiful, elegant and powerful tools for the pursuit of destiny.

PART 1

THE EIGHT EXTRAORDINARY VESSELS and the UNFOLDING OF JING

CHAPTER 1

ILLNESS AS A FORM OF COMMUNICATION

Human beings are designed with self-preservation in mind. The body has many ways in which it supports continued life. When we are running low on fluids we become thirsty. This thirst is a communication from the body that we need to increase our fluid intake. If we listen to the communication and have something to drink then the communication goes away. If we don't listen the communication gets louder.

The sleepiness we feel at the end of the day is our body's message that we need downtime in the form of sleep to restore. If we ignore that sleepiness and keep going then eventually we will become exhausted and sick.

Physical pain is our body's way of telling us that we are injured and we need to slow down and do what is needed to repair. If we slow down and attend to the injury or pain then the pain will eventually go away. If we refuse to slow down when we are injured then the injury worsens or the treatment becomes more complicated or invasive, which then may result in increased suffering.

Depression, anxiety or emotional instability is how we know we are living in an unbalanced way. It is the body's way of telling us we need to change how we are living our lives. The choices we make are not supporting the balance between body and mind.

Mental and emotional imbalances tell us that we are not living our purpose in the most authentic way possible.

Illness is our body's way of telling us that we are out of alignment with the natural order of our life. It suggests that our lifestyle choices or beliefs are not supporting the fullest expression of who we are.

This is not a rush to judgment or self-blame. I am not saying that people create every illness they suffer by making bad choices. Illness has many determining factors that may have little to do with daily lifestyle choices, including genetics and virulent pathogens. What I am saying is that every illness offers us a chance to learn and grow. We can use illness to peel away that which is not truly who we are. We can recognize illness as the body's way of trying to tell us we have something we need to learn in order to feel more whole, in order to be well.

There are people who are "cured" of diseases that never "heal" and there are those who are not cured but still know what it is to be whole and therefore are healed.

Somewhere along the passage of time, many of us have learned to ignore or override the communication of the body. We have somehow allowed our minds to disconnect from our bodies as if they are two separate entities. We have learned to keep going when we are hungry or thirsty or to go without adequate sleep even when we are so very tired. We have learned to keep eating long after we are full. We can no longer hear the communication that comes with being sated. We have even learned to hold our urine because it is just too inconvenient to make a trip to the bathroom.

Perhaps because we have ignored these basic forms of communication for so long we have become blind and deaf to some of the more subtle needs of the body and spirit. We have learned to ignore the needs of the body to move or to be outdoors in nature. We have been indoctrinated, especially in the US, to be satisfied with a few precious days of vacation, telling ourselves that job security is more important than our need to nourish our souls and recharge our vitality. We have learned to take two pills so that we can continue on without experiencing pain. We have learned that a glass of wine or a puff or two of marijuana can help us to forget the stress or pressures of the day. We self-medicate so that we can ignore the discomfort arising in our bodies as a result of that stress.

Those decisions to ignore or override the needs of the body and spirit come at a price. When we stop listening, the communication becomes louder and more serious. For instance, if we ignore the fact that we feel bad after we eat sugar and we continue to eat it, eventually the body communicates in a more serious fashion by producing stronger disruptions in insulin balance, which may lead to diabetes or insulin resistance and these diseases lead to many more, like cardiovascular disease, neurological disease and blindness. You do not suddenly develop Type 2 Diabetes. Long before you have this disease your body has been trying to tell you that something is not right. You do not suddenly get obstruction of your coronary arteries or tumors. The body has been talking to you all along, trying to get you to pay attention. The body will keep trying to get your attention. It will keep trying to get you to understand the communication.

It is human nature to avoid or resist change until our present circumstances are intolerable. Here is the big piece of the puzzle: the body, when directed by spirit, is perfectly capable of making the circumstances of life very intolerable. It can make us so miserable that we must change or die.

The communication usually begins as a whisper. That vague sense of unease. That feeling that all is not right. If we ignore that voice it will get louder. The innate intelligence of the body-mind will create symptoms that are uncomfortable or inconvenient. Woe unto those who ignore this voice or woe unto those who think they are fixing the problem by taking two pills to relieve the pain or an antidepressant to improve their mood, all the while continuing the behavior that the body-mind is rejecting. Eventually the symptoms will become so loud that it is as if some part of the whole goes on strike and sets up a picket line, shouting out its demands and refusing to budge until we negotiate in good faith.

How many times have you heard patients diagnosed with cancer or some other devastating illness say they knew something was wrong long before they were diagnosed? They have learned over time to ignore the little warnings, to override the voice. Maybe fear stops them from listening or maybe they are just too busy and they tell themselves they will get to it later. Many of us live in a culture that devalues the body's communication. We are trained to value achievement, accumulation or accolades at all costs. We are trained to push past our perceived limitations and conquer our weaknesses as we conquer the world around us. As the ads for Nike say: "Just do it."

The human system is directed by the need for homeostasis so that function can continue. Or more simply said, the body is driven by survival. The spirit, however, knows that survival may be important but is not enough. The spirit knows that life can have meaning and purpose. The spirit can and will create an environment where a tremendous amount of physical or emotional suffering can occur so that we will let go of our resistance and embrace the lessons we are here to learn.

Self-preservation is important too. The mechanisms for self-preservation are built into the body and they are important. The human spirit relies on this self-preservation in order to pursue its curriculum or purpose for being here. If we develop a good relationship with our bodies and we trust and respond appropriately to the communication the body provides, then it becomes easier to move beyond the need for survival. Once we can move beyond survival as our sole or primary driving force we can pursue the meaning and purpose that the heart desires.

This journey of self-discovery or self-awareness is the most healing process there is. To be able to recognize that nothing about the essence of who we truly are is ever damaged by the challenges and trauma in life is an empowering experience. For instance, a broken heart is indeed a painful experience that makes us doubt ourselves and may make us want to withdraw from the world. But learning to deal with loss and heal a broken heart is often the experience that helps us to develop compassion. A broken heart may be cracked and held together with spackle and chicken wire but those cracks shed the light of our indomitable spirit into the world. Hurt and sorrow, pain and shame have the potential to make us more fully who we are by whittling away the false skin or armor created by the need for self-preservation. If only we can be open to the communication and learn. If only we are willing to be vulnerable and experience those feelings without judgment but rather with the intent of embracing our humanness.

Chinese Medicine (CM) is uniquely suited to supporting the relationship between the body and the mind. This medicine has a long history of respect for the reality that the body and mind are one. There is an understanding that the physical body, the mental-emotional body and the spiritual body are inseparable. Humanity is the ongoing relationship between all of these aspects of humanness and the world around us.

In an effort to fit into a more allopathic (Western) medical approach, modern-day CM is often focused on alleviating the physical or emotional symptoms of suffering. It is very good at this. But, as a medical model it has so much more to offer. It is a system that has its basis in the understanding that wellness comes from living in accordance with the natural order of things. That means that the philosophical underpinnings of CM have an appreciation for the balance of yin and yang and living with respect for the changes of light and dark, hot and cold, dry and wet that come with seasonal change. It also recognizes that we must develop consciousness about how we use our resources to fulfill our purpose for being here. We must be aware of how our thoughts, beliefs and actions impact our physical well-being.

There are many systems in CM, some of which are not even Chinese, and many different approaches to take using those systems. For me, the one that is most effective in helping people with issues around suffering and self-preservation is the Eight Extraordinary Vessels (8 EV). These vessels are unique in that they alone are prenatal in nature. They impact the development of our humanity during gestation before we take our first breath. There are said to be "outside" or "separate" from the rest of the system. They are vessels of essence and they carry with them, from the previous generation (or incarnation), all that is needed for our journey to unfold. As we will see in later chapters, each of these vessels has a unique function that helps us to adapt to the big challenges of life. It is these same challenges, when met with resistance, that may cause the greatest suffering.

SUFFERING

What is the nature of suffering? Is it part of the pain complex or is it something altogether different? Is suffering always present when there is pain? Does suffering cause pain or pain cause suffering? We could probably engage in a lengthy conversation about the definition or semantics of the word suffering. It is a complex theme.

After pondering these questions for a while, I prefer to think of pain and suffering as being separate but often associated. Let us say, for the sake of conversation, that pain is something that can be identified as a specific sensation in the body. It can be derived from physical injury or illness or evoked by emotional imbalance. It is, in CM, a sensation that arises from stagnation or lack of movement. Pain is a form of communication that the body produces in order to get our attention. Suffering, on the other hand, is our relationship to the sensation of pain. The quote that is often wrongly attributed to the Buddha: "pain is inevitable, suffering is optional," provides a valuable distinction between the two. One cannot live without experiencing pain. It is an essential part of living. It is the feedback we need to learn from our experiences. As children we learn that when we touch the stove or a fire we get burned. The pain of the burn teaches us to use caution when approaching things that are hot.

Suffering can also be useful in learning. In fact, many people can override their ability to learn from the sensation of pain and have difficulty learning from pain if it is not accompanied by some type of suffering. In gyms all over the country the rallying call to fitness used to be "no pain, no gain." So people seeking fitness, weight loss or even just a six-pack to impress were risking serious injury by overcoming the pain signals and driving towards their goal. Imagine embracing pain until it creates so much suffering that you have to listen. Of course, by then you may be on crutches for a few months or you may need rotator cuff surgery. So in that sense, we may need a certain amount of suffering to insure that the communication of the body is heard, understood and stored away for future reference. It becomes a memory that we can call up to give us a context for similar experiences. We learn from our pain and suffering.

More often than not, lingering suffering may be an impediment to moving forward. The emotional quality of our suffering can keep us focused on the pain. Sometimes even after the pain is gone we have fear of the pain recurring, so the suffering continues. When this happens it may eventually prohibit us from being able to see the possibility of learning, growing and healing or the suffering may make it difficult to have hope for a future that exists without anticipation of injury or the misery that accompanies it.

So much of the pain we experience is emotional in nature. Even when it begins with physical pain we often experience uncomfortable emotions related to that pain. We become angry, frustrated, worried, afraid or sad about the pain or the event that led to the pain. Just as when we get our feelings hurt it produces a sensation of physical discomfort in the chest or abdomen, so too will physical pain cause us to experience an emotional response to that pain. So, then the question arises: "What is our relationship to our emotions?" Can we accept them as part of our human experience? Feelings may be useful feedback from the body/mind that allow us to recognize the fullness of life's experiences. Even more importantly, accepting that emotions are only one part of a very complex and elegant system of communication allows us to give them their due without being run by them.

Some people value their feelings above their intellect. They may feel as though their feelings are sacred, valuable and more in alignment with their innate nature. When I was younger and on a mission of self-discovery, one of the most profound things a therapist said to me was: "They are just your feelings." At first I was affronted. "What do you mean, *they are just my feelings*? How could you minimize my feelings? I am a person who has deep feelings." My feelings were precious to me and I valued them and the information they brought me. Of course, with that information came suffering that over the years lead me to hole up in my bedroom and read ten books a week, cowering in a corner of my bed hoping the rest of the world would just go away. Over time I began to realize that what the therapist was trying to tell me was that my feelings are not who I am. They are something I am experiencing and I have a choice about how I experience them. I do not need to ignore them or over value them. I just need to place them in balance with the rest of my experiences.

Emotions are information that we can choose to use for growth or not. Like all other forms of energy they are transitory, always changing. It is only our attachment to them or our resistance to experiencing them that keeps them in our field for a longer time. If we hold on to emotion or embody it as if it is ours, it goes against the laws of nature and that will result in suffering.

Many people are very uncomfortable with emotions. This may in part be cultural in nature or a by-product of our upbringing or it may be based on a person's previous experiences. For instance, many people who have a strong intellect are often more comfortable with "thinking" about a situation than dealing with it from an emotional perspective. They value logic over feelings or maybe they were expected to value logic over feelings when they were younger. Unfortunately, some experiences in life cannot be managed by intellect alone, especially when those experiences involve relationships. It is helpful to have an understanding of our own feelings if we are to appreciate the feelings of others. Far too often, thinkers lack empathy for themselves and others, which may affect their ability to have relationships that are productive and joyful. If they cannot deal with the uncomfortable experiences they cannot feel the positive emotions either.

Some people are out of touch with their feelings. Life may present us with so many situations that evoke strong feelings that we learn through self-preservation to turn down the volume on our emotional responses. We may become numb or distanced from our feelings. I have had many patients who inform me that they have anxiety or depression and when I ask them where they experience that in their bodies, they cannot tell me. They have lost touch with the container of their spirit. In fact, some have even looked confused when I ask the question as if they cannot even find a context for what I am asking. Perhaps they think that the feelings they are experiencing are a whole separate system that has nothing to do with the body they are inhabiting.

Emotions can be a very powerful tool and some people learn very early in life how to manipulate others by using their emotions. They may express their feelings in a very dramatic way to illicit a specific response from those around them. You might think of the "terrible twos" although as a mother I would hasten to say that the third year is actually worse. Regardless, at some point in their early development, children make an attempt to manipulate their parents and get what they want by dropping to the ground and howling like they have been stabbed. They learn quickly that this is most effective when it is done in public. An audience buys support and places pressure on the parent to end the conflict quickly, even if it means giving in. When my son was small, I made the mistake of taking him to the grocery store during the "meltdown hour." This is the time of the day when children who have skipped their naps start to short-circuit in a way that is predictable and yet still disconcerting. I should have known better but the cupboards were bare and dinner time was soon arriving. He was being difficult, as is typical of tired and hungry children. I was short-tempered and frustrated, which is typical of tired and hungry mothers. I was running out of patience and I snapped at him and told him to stop it. At which point he burst into tears, sobbing as if the sorrow produced by my loss of patience was coming from the depth of his very soul and then he proceeded to say, loudly enough so that several other shoppers could hear: "I'm sorry Mommy, please don't hit me, I'll be a good boy." Well, it will be of no surprise to many of you that his emotional display worked. I picked him up, left the cart in the aisles and took my child and my mortification out to the car and went home, all the while wondering if Child Protective Services would be following me home. It is, I believe, a rite of passage and another opportunity for parents to learn how to parent. Our children are our most important teachers. If at that time in my life I had had a healthier relationship to my feelings I would have known that my fatigue, frustration and sense of overwhelm were being mirrored by my son and we would have never left the house. It would have been a good night to have food delivered and after a warm bath, to cuddle on the couch and read stories. If my relationship to my feelings was healthier, I would have been listening to the communication from my body that said: "I am tired, I am less resilient, I am not in a good frame of mind because I need food and sleep."

Should you have a relationship with someone who is 25 or older and they are still throwing tantrums or using emotions to get what they want, then you are dealing with someone who has an unhealthy relationship to their feelings. Your response to that manipulation can also be a measure of your relationship to your emotions. If our relationship to our feelings is unhealthy then we are assured of a certain amount of suffering. Also, if the people around us have trouble dealing with their emotions then their suffering may spread to those nearest and often dearest and this will trigger the suffering of all involved. "If Momma ain't happy, nobody is happy."

For emotions to be valuable for growth we must remember we are not our grief. We are not our anger. We are not our fear. To take it a step further, those emotions are not even really ours; they are an energy that exists regardless of whether we are unable to experience or acknowledge them. We may not know we are angry, we may not be able to feel it, but that will not stop those around us from experiencing us as angry even if we don't. Most of us have had the experience of being in a room with someone who is not aware of how angry or sad they are. Their lack of awareness leads to an inability to take responsibility for their emotion and that emotion is then spewed onto everyone else in the room. It can be very uncomfortable to be on the receiving end of this, especially if we are unable to deal with our own emotions. If, however, we can recognize that we are experiencing a certain emotion then we can take responsibility for it and deal with the problem that the emotional communication is trying to bring to our attention.

Culture and upbringing may also predispose us to suffering. We are imprinted with a certain relationship to suffering depending on how we are raised. Some people may be raised with the principle of original sin. They may believe that they deserve to suffer, just for being born. They may have been taught to believe that suffering strengthens their relationship to G-d. Others may believe that suffering is a symptom of wrong-doing and a sign that G-d is displeased with us. Still others may believe that suffering has nothing to do with G-d and it is something we choose. We may have been taught by example that suffering is noble and our ability to endure it makes us a better person. The significance of all of this is not about who is right or wrong about suffering but rather that it is important to be conscious of how those early principles imprint on us and affect our relationship to suffering.

Long time sufferers may become very attached to their suffering, especially if they believe that suffering is noble. There is often a resistance to change because change means letting go of the past, letting go of our emotions, letting go of our unhealthy perspectives. This is not unlike Stockholm Syndrome in which hostages will express empathy or sympathy towards their captors, identifying with or defending them. This is a traumatic form of bonding and it is theorized that this allows the captive to deal with the threat of captivity. Emotions and suffering can hold us captive. When people become attached to their suffering it is as if they are saying: "I agree with this suffering. This is my suffering; no one else can understand it. My suffering is noble and has meaning."

This attachment allows them to find some meaning in the suffering. I see this often in patients who have chronic unremitting pain or loss of a limb or even those undergoing chemotherapy or radiation. This is not to say that these people are feeling sorry for themselves; it is much more complex than that. They have had the rug pulled out from under their feet. The trauma that has brought them to this place has been serious enough that their normal coping mechanism is insufficient to protect them from the suffering. They are struggling to make sense of what is happening to them. They may want to go back to the way things used to be but they know that will never happen so they invest in a new norm. They invest in their suffering.

For these patients to get back on track to pursuing their destiny they need to let go of their attachment to their suffering. We can help them to experience the truth that their wholeness of spirit and authenticity are not reliant on the perfection of their physical form. We are more than our feelings, more than our suffering. There is a part of us that is at the core of who we really are that has never suffered. We can be whole, feel whole and live from that place even when we are in pain. Even when we have suffered.

RESISTANCE TO CHANGE

It is human nature to respond to pain by leaning away from it and going into the past to a time when we were comfortable. The desires we have to be pain-free are based on our history. This means we want a future that is a replication of a more comfortable time in our past. "I just want it to be the way it used to be." This desire, although natural, ignores or devalues the message (pain) in the here and now that is offering us an opportunity to change.

I have seen a number of patients who develop some type of recurring pain in their 40s and 50s. Maybe they have knee pain or some recurring back pain. Very often, their response to that pain is: "This never used to happen to me in my 30s. I am not doing anything different so why is this happening to me?" I hear patient say things like: "I've been lifting this same weight for years, why is it causing a problem now?" The answer of course is that you are not the same as you were 20 years ago. It is not just that you are older, it is also that everything about your life is different. Maybe you have a sedentary job now. Maybe you have two kids and you don't get enough sleep. Maybe you have a mortgage that places a financial stress on you. What matters is not what you could do in the past. What matters is that your body is trying to tell you that it needs you to change. It has probably been trying to tell you that for years in many small ways and now it has had enough and it is speaking louder.

Some patients will try to avoid the message by leaning into the future. "I'm over this, I just want to be on the other side of it." This perspective also devalues the message of pain. Patients in this state are not in the present moment and they are trying to propel themselves into a future where the pain never happened. In order to avoid suffering they are often trying to "bypass" the message. My mother battled metastatic breast cancer for many years. She had very powerful "suffering-bypass" skills. She was raised in Scotland at the end of WWII when rationing was still the norm. Life was not easy and she learned, as all of us Scots do, to pull herself up by her bootstraps and get on with it. She was raised to stop dwelling on what was not available or to ignore what was uncomfortable. She was taught to ignore that which could not be changed. When she was first diagnosed she was terrified, but true to her upbringing she did get on with it. On the day of her surgery, she was admitted to the hospital at 6:00 am, had a modified radical mastectomy, which included the removal of several lymph nodes, and by noon that very same day she was ensconced in the recliner at home, bandaged and bruised with drains coming out of her chest, looking for something to eat. Even though she was pea green and in obvious pain, life was moving on for her. Her resilience was awe-inspiring. When I told her that I had found some local cancer support groups for her, she looked at me like I was the Village Idiot (her words not mine) and said: "Why would I want to be around sick people?"

Her first metastases was to her brain. Tumor removed, moving on. Just like the last time. The cancer did finally take her many years later when it spread to her bones. She never really let it stop her, which is good, right? When I look back on that time I wonder if she had been available to the lessons of self-care that many cancer patients learn, might she have lived longer? Might she have lived with less pain? I wonder if she had faced her mortality and dread of dying would that have changed her experience? I also can't help but wonder how I would approach the same set of circumstances. I have worked for over 25 years now to try to learn those lessons in the hope that my body will not need to have the same experience.

It is often difficult to recognize resistance, as it can take many forms. It may be active or passive, overt or covert. Active or overt resistance is easier to see because it is direct. The resistance is strong. There is visible tension, palpable anger, bitterness, resentment. The patient often has hyperactive boundaries (touchy) and may be prone to justice seeking (someone deserves to pay for this). Passive or covert resistance is a little bit trickier to spot. Passive resistance comes from lack of resources. The patient is too tired to carry on. There is visible collapse and evidence of defeat and surrender to victimization. The patient may be prone to seeking sympathy and have weak boundaries. In covert resistance, patients tell you they put in their best effort but despite their efforts something always happens to prevent them from doing what they must. This looks like attempted compliance but nothing changes. This occurs when people do not have the will to change but don't want to be judged by others. "I am really trying." "I just can't seem to manage to take the midday dose of herbs." Resistance to change in any of its forms, overt or covert, can lead to suffering.

For some, much of their life is infused with great or consistent suffering. Who knows why that is true for some more than others? There do seem to be some common characteristics in patients who have prolonged suffering. They include: fear of the unknown, a sense of unworthiness, guilt, shame, anger (in all of its many forms) and craving or desire (desperately wanting something you do not currently have). It is also very common for patients who have lingering suffering to have a history of trauma or mental-emotional disorders like anxiety, depression or addiction. These issues may cause the suffering to linger or overwhelm the patient and this will also complicate the diagnosis and treatment. When you are treating a patient who is suffering you are often treating their history. Not just the physical history of the condition but also their emotional history, their character style, their self-defense mechanism. It can be challenging to weave together all the parts of the patient's story to create a context for the patient's current reality.

Context for the suffering can be addressed at the same time one treats the pain. We can create a treatment that helps patients to accept the current reality. Until patients are fully present to what is, there is little likelihood of permanent change. We can create a treatment that instills hope and confidence that change is possible. We are able to give our patients the ability to conceive of a new way of being. We can support their ability to transform. We can support their ability to let go and finally to reconnect with their authentic sense of self. We can do that at the same time we are treating the pain.

This is where the Eight Extraordinary Vessels (8 EV) shine. The unique nature of these vessels allows us to treat the current complaint in conjunction with the resistance and beliefs that hinder growth.

CM has an "inner tradition" which recognizes that medicine can be used as a tool to aid in spiritual development. Physical, emotional and mental illness is directly correlated to the degree to which an individual is capable of living his/her destiny. There is some evidence of this in both the classic literature of CM and the current literature of acupuncture, metaphysics and psychological disciplines.

Using the 8 EV helps to create a treatment plan that facilitates consciousness and increases awareness. This then changes how results or success are measured. Progress is typically measured in increased awareness of self, improved coping mechanisms, mature responses to emotional difficulty, healthier relationships and a renewed sense of purpose. Of course this usually also means that the treatment will lead to a decrease of physical pain and suffering but this by no means is the primary focus.

To understand the 8 EV you need to understand their place in the channel system. This can best be understood from the perspective of the levels of qi. Each level of qi in the body is affected by a different system. There are three levels: wei, ying and yuan.

Wei qi or protective qi, as it is sometimes known, governs the surface of the body. The surface of the body is governed by the six cutaneous zones and the sinew channels. These channels do not have a direct connection to the organs. That means their response to the outside world is pre-thought. It is instinctive and reflexive and because they do not have a connection to the organ function their function does not require cognition or consciousness. When you are exposed to exterior pathogenic factors the wei qi responds before you can say to yourself: "I feel like I am coming down with something. Maybe I should activate my wei qi." If you hear a loud noise you will flinch or duck long before cognition of what that noise might be kicks in. "What was that?" comes after the flinch.

As we move inward to the ying qi level what we see is the influence of the blood on process and function. Ying qi or nutritive qi is the qi aspect of blood. This level is governed by the function of the luo-collaterals and the primary channels. There is a clear connection to the organ function and therefore to cognition. These two systems are essential to postnatal processing. Here we are dealing with emotions as they relate to the daily events of life or the relationships in our everyday existence. At this level the functions of the heart, pericardium and spleen have an important job to do in how we mediate emotions and what lifestyle choices we make.

When you start to look at the constitutional aspects of health you are looking a little deeper into the channel system. You are reaching into the yuan qi (source qi) level. This level is influenced by the divergent or distinct meridians. The Divergent Meridians are said to extend the influence of the primary channel system into a deeper level. The nature of this system strengthens the relationship between yuan qi and wei qi.

Since jing is yuan qi in its densest form we can also see the influence of the 8 EV at this level. Since they are by nature jing vessels they are a deep expression of the constitution, and their prenatal nature allows us to impact the patient's relationship to their curriculum. They give us a window into belief systems, healthy or not. They give us insight about a person's relationship to Self. They help us to understand how trauma might limit growth and development and they allow us to see where genetics, lineage and early childhood experiences shape our personality and our way of adapting to evolutionary stress.

If you want to help to ease a patient's suffering that can be achieved at any level but if you want to help a person become more of who they are so that they are less vulnerable to suffering you need the 8 EV. If you want to help a person to let go of deep-seated beliefs that are impeding their ability to grow, gain mastery of themselves and pursue their curriculum with meaning and purpose then you need the 8 EV. If a patient has an acute sprain you can ease a person's suffering by treating the appropriate sinew channels but if a patient has chronic pain that directly reflects their inability to manage their lives then the sinew channel will not have the same impact as the 8 EV.

CHAPTER 2

THE EIGHT EXTRAORDINARY VESSELS (8 EV)

aka: Qi Jing Ba Mai, The Eight Ancestral Channels,
The Eight Prenatal Vessels, The Eight Psychic Channels

The name of these vessels implies that they are different from the 12 primary channels. They are the original vessels that are present in-utero during gestation. They engage the genetic material passed down from one generation to the next and they are responsible for how the fetus develops. Although they are the root of the 12 primary channels they do not have a direct connection to the internal organs. They are a separate system that influences the primary channels because they store and distribute yuan qi and jing throughout the body. The 8 EV can be seen as the reservoirs of vital substances that support physiological function. Up until the moment of birth these are the only active vessels. They contain within them all that you have been given through your parents and the care you received during the time you were in the womb. They are the basis for your constitution and are linked to the function of the kidneys, which are the repository of jing.

GENERATIONAL TRANSMISSION

The 8 EV are vessels of curriculum. They contain within them the primary resources you have been given for your journey through life. They regulate the seven/eight year cycles of growth and development. They are broad band vessels that influence all levels of qi from the wei qi on the surface to the deepest aspect of yuan qi. They support the body during transition and they help us to be adaptable in the face of change, especially when that transition is evolutionary in nature. When a transition affects who we are and who we are trying to become then the 8 EV are involved. In some ways you can think of these vessels like the Holy Grail. They sustain life and supply us with what we need to continue living. On the other hand, they contain not only the genetic strengths passed on to us from previous generations but also the weakness and traumas experienced in those generations. These genetic strengths and weaknesses become part of our curriculum in life and they may be the basis for many of our unconscious or limiting beliefs. If a person experiences a trauma that cannot be resolved in their lifetime (for instance some Holocaust survivors) then that trauma is stored in the bones (jing), which is then passed down to the next generation. We are not our parents but we carry their strengths and weaknesses and those of many previous generations. This generational information can be a gift or a burden. It can be the determining factor in how we live our lives and it can be the stimulus we need to change. This generational information can imbue us with a belief system that supports our growth and development or in some cases it can create a template for unsupportive beliefs. When we are weighed down by the experiences of previous generations, life may seem more difficult. The effort required to overcome those beliefs can be exhausting. We may find ourselves unable to sustain the changes we make in life because of the burdens of previous generations. For lasting change to occur you may need to find a way to address the imprinting of this prenatal level of being-ness. The 8 EV can help us to bring into consciousness the impact of this generational transmission, for when we can see it, we can choose whether or not we want to continue to live our lives through that history.

THE CURIOUS ORGANS

These vessels have a direct link with the six curious organs (six extraordinary fu). They influence these curious organs in ways that the primary channels cannot. The brain is regulated by the Du Mai, Yin Qiao and Yang Qiao. The uterus is regulated by the Ren Mai and the Chong Mai. The blood vessels are regulated by the Chong Mai. The Gall Bladder is regulated by the Dai Mai. The marrow is regulated by the Chong Mai and Du Mai and the bones are regulated by the Chong and Ren. This means that the 8 EV have a direct influence on the organs and tissues responsible for transformation occurring through circulation, growth, development and procreation.

THE ORIFICES

The 8 EV are also closely linked to the orifices of the body. The sensory orifices of the head (eyes, ears, nose and mouth) are how we take the outside world in and the lower orifices are how we let the world go through urination, defecation and ejaculation. Through the orifices, the 8 EV negotiate the sensory experiences of life. These days there is an overwhelming amount of sensory stimulation and the 8 EV must work overtime in order to process that information and in some cases protect us from the sheer volume of it all. I sometimes ponder the reasons for the increase of complex digestive syndromes in the modern world. It seems as if the increase in this sensory input puts a tremendous burden on the digestive and elimination systems. The creation of supposed advances in agriculture, pesticides, antibiotics, preservatives and petrochemicals stress the system that is supposed to help us to adapt. The evolutionary stress of all this new input has made it more difficult to transform. The 8 EV have a powerful impact on how we receive and how we let go, physiologically, emotionally and spiritually. We can use them to help our patients and ourselves deal with all of this sensory input. We can use them to help us digest life with more consciousness and we can use them to help us let go of that which is no longer in alignment with our pursuit of meaning and purpose.

EVOLUTIONARY STRESS

These 8 EV become activated by evolutionary stress. That is the physical stress of evolution and also the mental-emotional and spiritual stress of evolution. They become active when there is a dire need for change. These vessels are the driving force behind our reasons for being here.

DESTINY AND CURRICULUM

To make use of these vessels as fully as possible one must understand their connection to destiny or curriculum. At the moment of conception, jing from both parents is combined creating the potential for new life. The Heavenly Mandate is bestowed and with it the seed of potential is planted. This potential is the foundation of life unfolding or one might say it is the source of our curriculum in life. We have been gifted with all that we need to fulfill our life's journey. If we pursue that journey with authenticity then we are moving wholeheartedly towards our Destiny. If we move away from authenticity into a lesser or created self then we are laying down to fate. To live our Destiny we align ourselves with the will of Heaven. For all you atheists out there who are shuddering at the thought of aligning yourself with some place in the clouds (Heaven), you can think of it this way: to fulfill your destiny in life you must align yourself with the nature of the universe. To do this it helps to have an understanding of: Who? Why? What? Who am I? Why am I here? What am I doing about it?

When we are in the womb we are under the influence of Pre-Heaven/prenatal qi. In this prenatal existence we are gifted this potential and during the gestational time it is up to our mothers to nourish this potential to the best of their ability. Once we are born, we fall under the influence of Post-Heaven/postnatal qi. Life has its challenges and these challenges impact how we live in the world. If we can face these challenges while maintaining our sense of who we are then we will be pursuing our curriculum authentically. If we forget who we are or if we lose our connection to our Self, then it is easier to lay down to fate and feel the burden of our unfulfilled curriculum.

The 8 EV are the vessels that link us to that curriculum and to our original nature. They can help us to remember who we are and why we are here and they can provide resources to get back on our path to pursuing our Destiny. They give us a deep connection to the very essence of who we are and allow for our jing to unfold in a way that brings it into the light of shen/spirit.

NATURE OF THE INDIVIDUAL VESSELS

Each of these vessels has its own pathway, function and relationship to vital substances. The Ren and Du Mai have their own points and the rest of the 8 EV share points on the primary channels. They each have a master point that is like a key in a lock that opens the door to that vessel. Sometimes we use couple points to support the function of the vessel but that is by no means required.

Vessel	Vital substance	Master	Couple
Chong Mai	Sea of Blood, Sea of Yuan Qi, Sea of the Five Zang and Six Fu, Sea of the 12 Primary Channels	Sp-4	Pc-6
Ren Mai	Sea of Yin	Lu-7	Ki-6
Du Mai	Sea of Yang	SI-3	UB-62
Dai Mai	Sea of Ming Men	GB-41	SJ-5
Yin Wei	Links blood/yin and the interior	Pc-6	Sp-4
Yin Qiao	Removes accumulation from the abdomen (yin)	Ki-6	Lu-7
Yang Qiao	Removes accumulation from the head (yang)	UB-62	SI-3
Yang Wei	Links qi and the exterior	SJ-5	GB-41

MASTER POINTS

The master points of the 8 EV were not part of the original discussions in the classics. These master points were added later as a means of focusing or directing the treatment to a particular vessel. There is no definitive explanation for why the specific points were chosen but there are some interesting facts to ponder.

For instance, four out of the eight master points are also luo-collateral points. This gives us some idea of the resonance between the 8 EV and the luo-collateral system. Both systems have a profound connection to blood and healthy circulation. From the perspective of suffering this means that these vessels can powerfully impact emotional processing, the need for self-preservation and our capacity to adapt in the face of change. Both systems have a networking function that allows them to make both deeper and more superficial connections. Because of this, both systems have a broader impact than the primary channel system. Both systems have a regulating effect on the polarity of yin and yang. The luo-collaterals balance yin and yang in the limbs and the 8 EV balance polarity in the trunk. They are both very effective in help us to let go of that which no longer serves.

Two of the master points are not actually master points (UB-62, Ki-6). They are in fact the first points on their associated pathways. This might imply that the Qiao vessels really are more closely related to the primary system than the other vessels. We might think of them as conduits between the primary channels and the 8 EV.

YIN, YANG AND THE FORMATION OF LIFE

Since the 8 EV are vessels of curriculum or ancestral vessels one might also think of the master points as directly reflecting the formation of life as it is represented by the movement in the cycles of yin and yang.

Shao yang: GB-41, SJ-5

The energy of shao yang/lesser yang is where the impulse for life begins. It is the beginning of yang, the first spark of life. The energy here is like the seed sprouting and pushing its way up through the soil into the sunlight. It is the energy of Wood, the energy of spring, the energy of emergence or birth.

Tai yang: UB-62, SI-3

The energy of tai yang/greater yang is about yang reaching its peak. This is the energy of Fire and it is the fullest expression of yang. This is the energy of peak growth. It represents the fullest function of the motive force of yang. From here the energy begins to turn towards yin.

Shao yin: Ki-6, Pc-6[1]

The energy of shao yin/lesser yin is about discharge or release. This is the energy of Metal, which is the energy of letting go. We know who were are and we are ready to let go of that which no longer serves us. We spend the first half of our lives gathering things, accumulating things so that we may learn and grow. We are in effect collecting stuff. Eventually we then turn towards letting go of that which we have collected. Refining, reducing, cutting away the fat or freeing up the stagnation that comes with accumulation.

Tai yin: Sp-4, Lu-7

The energy of tai yin/greater yin is the energy of withdrawal, dormancy and hibernation. It is the extreme of yin as it is expressed through Water. As we are nearing the end of our lives we begin to pull back and become more introspective. There is a conservation of resources as we reflect on what is most essential. So this reflects the deepest aspect of who we are and holds our deepest truths.

These energies are reflected throughout a whole life but they are also expressed every day in the cycles of yang and yin, waking and sleeping. When we look at this cyclic process it at least can give us some theory to help us understand why these points may have been chosen as master points of the vessels that govern the cycles of life.

---

1   Here Pc-6 replaces the heart point that might have been chosen, because it is more respectful to treat the Emperor through its minister or protector.

CLINICAL USE OF THE EIGHT EXTRAORDINARY VESSELS

The typical use in a clinical setting is to combine two of the vessels together to access a sea of energy with a way to transport that energy. This is sometimes called nuclear pairing. These pairs work together to influence a specific area of the body.

Sea	Area of influence	Transporter
Ren Mai	Abdomen, chest, lungs, throat and face	Yin Qiao
Du Mai	Posterior aspect of the body, spine, neck, head, eyes and brain	Yang Qiao
Chong Mai	Inner aspect of legs, stomach, heat, chest and abdomen	Yin Wei
Dai Mai	Lateral aspect of the legs and body, shoulders, lateral aspect of the neck and retro-auricular region	Yang Wei

This is by no means the only way to look at these vessels. As is true with all channel theory, the trajectories/pathways of the 8 EV are informative. If you want to understand these vessels more deeply and use them more effectively you must know where they begin, where they end and where they travel in between. This can take some time and patience but it is definitely worth it.

You could of course decide to use the Yin Wei for a patient who has anxiety based on symptomology of palpitations, chest pain and blood deficiency. But if you know the trajectory of the vessel and the points along the way you will have a much deeper understanding of how to use that vessel in a more directed and powerful manner. The channel pathway is more important than any individual point on the channel.

The Chong Mai for instance has five distinct branches and each branch has a specific impact on pathology in the Chong. If you know these branches then you can treat just one branch or you can support a relationship between two or more branches in your treatment.

In understanding the trajectories of each vessel you can see pathology in the 8 EV based on posture and demeanor as well. For example, you can see the influence of the Yang Qiao in those people who are over-extended in the world, driving forward all of the time and never stopping to smell the roses. They often have a very tense, upright posture and even their visual focus is often forward directed (tunnel vision/tai yang). The Yang Wei on the other hand often presents with a posture that has some twists and turns in it. The effort to adapt to life over time can often cause the structure to try to accommodate life's uncomfortable experiences by bracing in a way that affects rotation. These people also have difficulty turning the head and neck so that they can see their options. We can see both of these tendencies in the pathways.

There will be an image provided in each of the coming chapters for the individual vessels. This will allow you to see the pathway while reading about the functions and indications for its use. The visual will help you to see the reason that these vessels can do what they do.

For instance, it is meaningful that the Chong, Ren and Du Mai originate in the same area of the body. It is significant that this area of the lower burner, where they originate, is governed by the kidneys. These three channels are known as the "first ancestry" because they are the source vessels for all of the rest, just as the kidneys are the source vessels of postnatal existence because they are responsible for storing jing/essence.

It is also notable that the Yin and Yang Qiao begin in the regions of the heels/ankles and intersect at the eyes. These intersected pathways make it possible to view these two vessels as informing "stance" and "perspective." They connect us to the present moment in time and dictate how we see ourselves and the world around us. They influence how we take a stand.

The Yang Qiao and Yang Wei have points in common that intersect where the arms and the legs attach to the trunk and these two vessels govern action/locomotion (SI-10 and GB-29).

The pathway of the Dai Mai is the only horizontal vessel. It comes in contact with all of the other vessels and this helps to explain the integrating and harmonizing functions of this vessel. It is also said to have a stabilizing effect on the other vessels, just like a belt or girdle. Once again we can see the influence of the vessel directly through its trajectory.

There is no real need to think of these simply as pairs of channels used together to impact a specific area or function of the body. These vessels can be used individually with a single master point or they can be combined in ways not prescribed by the nuclear pairing. More simply said, you can mix and match. To mix and match effectively you must know the pathways of these vessels.

INDICATIONS FOR USE

Because the 8 EV are jing vessels they can be used to treat any problem that is related to the seven/eight year cycles of growth and development or any problems that affect the yuan qi or constitution. This would include the following.

- **Fertility issues**: recurring miscarriage, infertility, impotence, seminal issues, inability to achieve orgasm, vulvodynia and any gynecological condition that impacts fertility. These conditions are the cause for much suffering. The inability to procreate has a terrible impact on one's sense of self.

- **Developmental and congenital issues**: birth defects, epilepsy, babies born to addicted mothers and diseases that affect development like meningitis. Although we cannot change chromosomal abnormalities, the 8 EV can definitely improve how those congenital issues unfold, allowing the patient to have the best possible relationship to them. Many of the 8 EV have pathways that enter the brain so they can regulate neurological function, which in turn affects how we develop physically, emotionally and cognitively.

- **Pathology in the curious organs**: brain, uterus, bones, marrow, spine, blood vessels, gall bladder and prostate. Unlike the primary channel system, the 8 EV has a direct connection to these organs and tissues.

- **Diseases or conditions that affect the DNA**: aging and dying, cancer, AIDS and genetic disorders. Once again we are speaking of how jing unfolds. How do we feel about aging? Are we frightened of dying? How does having HIV/AIDS affect a person's sense of self? Can we make the most out of a life that begins with a genetic condition?

- **Psychological or emotional issues**: especially those that develop in the first cycle of jing (seven/eight years), including birth trauma, abandonment, abuse, neglect and illness or physical trauma, especially trauma or illness serious enough to require hospitalization. Those traumatic experiences leave an imprint on the psyche that may disrupt how our jing unfolds. We can help patients to renegotiate whether or not those experiences interfere with their pursuit of meaning and purpose. Even though we cannot change a person's history we can indeed help them to let go of the suffering associated with early trauma. When we are able to let go of the suffering then we are less likely to live our lives through the lens of that trauma. We may even be able to understand, at least a little, how that experience may have given us the opportunity to become more of who we are.

- **Unresolved conflict associated with identity**: suffering associated with gender, culture or sexual orientation. These are jing issues. When these issues create suffering then we are unable to fully accept who we are. Or perhaps we have suffering based on the fact that we may live in a society that makes us feel as though who we are is somehow unacceptable.

The list of physical, emotional or spiritual disorders that can be treated by the 8 EV goes on and on. What is key here is that the 8 EV can be used to support patients with any condition that is challenging their ability to maintain a connection to who they truly are. They are powerful advocates for those who are suffering because they can help patients to recognize that although they may feel lost, those feelings and the suffering associated with them in no way damage who they are at the core. Their original self is intact and all they need do is remember who they are, why they are here and what they are going to do about it. They remind us of the uniqueness and perfection of our original self and they allow us to once again bring forth the light that is our purpose for being here. The 8 EV can put us back on track to pursuing our destiny. When the 8 EV are functioning freely we can be the best of who we are, accepting that our current circumstances are an opportunity to learn, grow and become.

PRECAUTIONS

Opening the 8 EV is serious business. It must be handled with great respect and humility. If patients are not ready to do the work they may feel pressured or violated, which will cause them to further shut down. One should move into the 8 EV lightly with the idea of not trying to do too much at first. We want to give patients an opportunity to embrace the treatments and to open to the possibility that their suffering can be alleviated.

For this reason I personally prefer not to use the 8 EV in children in their first two cycles of jing unless there are severe congenital issues or diseases causing great suffering. For me, it is more respectful to let the curriculum of children unfold in the most natural way possible. So for most children I will try everything else first before turning to the 8 EV.

Another thing that is very important in the use of the 8 EV is the humility the practitioner brings to the treatment. It is important to create an environment with the treatment where patients have the opportunity to choose. We should not thrust our own agenda on the patient. This means we must provide the best treatment possible but not be attached to the outcome. It is hubris to assume we know what will put this patient back on track to pursuing their destiny or even that the return to that pursuit will look a certain way. I try my best to see my patients as unbroken. If I can see past their suffering to that wholeness that is untouched by present circumstance I feel as if I create a treatment that will balance the need to relieve suffering with an acknowledgement of their unique and perfect spirit.

A last word on cautions. These vessels are miraculous in their broad-reaching effect and they can basically treat anything. Just because they can doesn't mean you should. The 8 EV can be used to treat the common cold but doing that is like killing a fly with a cannon. It will get the job done but it is a terrible waste of resources. One must have a respect for the preciousness of jing and yuan qi. This is the deepest level of a person's existence. You have the knowledge to treat these lesser conditions with other systems and herbal formulations. With respect, use the 8 EV when you can be certain that the problem lies with yuan qi and jing. Use the 8 EV when you can determine that a patient's suffering is impeding their ability to express themselves fully in the world and is obstructing the pursuit of their destiny in a wholehearted fashion.

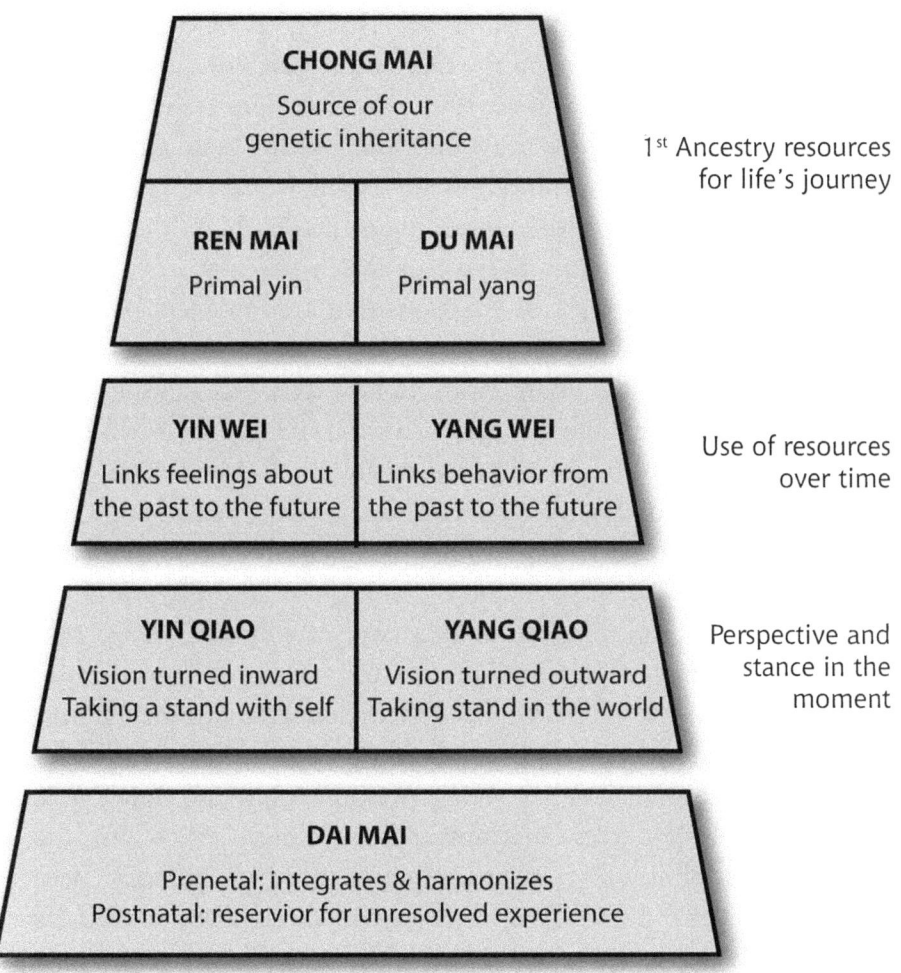

Figure 2.1: Development of the psyche

DEVELOPMENT OF THE PSYCHE

For the sake of our discussion about suffering, I prefer to view these 8 EV the way that I learned from Jeffrey Yuen. For me, this view explains the development of the psyche and how we grow, learn and individuate. In this view, the Chong Mai is the source of all of the other vessels. It gives birth to primal yin (Ren) and primal yang (Du). From the gifts of this first ancestry we must learn over time how to use our resources (Yin and Yang Wei) and we must eventually individuate and take a stand in who were are and how we see the world (Yin and Yang Qiao). At the end of this unfolding is the Dai Mai. It can serve to integrate the whole process or it can serve as an overflow vessel for those events or emotions that are too overwhelming to process.

This perspective allows us to see how resistance develops and to recognize the coping mechanisms that people use when they are under stress. It also makes it possible to understand how the environment or circumstances during our first cycle of jing (first seven/eight years) is responsible for much of what occurs later in our lives. The first ancestry (Chong, Du and Ren) unfolds during gestation through the first two years of life. During this time trauma, neglect and disease can negatively impact our resources. As we transition from the first ancestry of the Chong, Ren and Du we can begin to see not only the impact that early postnatal experiences have on our resources but also how a lack of prenatal resources (weakness in the Chong, Ren or Du) can affect our ability to face the challenges of a postnatal existence. We know that in the first cycle of jing (seven/eight years) children typically have a weaker digestive system. Their capacity for postnatal processing is affected by this weakness in the middle. They also do not have fully developed cognitive function. Their prefrontal cortex governing executive function is not yet fully developed so they must rely on the constitutional strength of the 8 EV. If during this time they suffer trauma, illness, rejection or abandonment then this will imprint deeply on the 8 EV. This imprint often defines how we make our way in the world as adults.

This way of organizing the 8 EV allows us to see the unfolding of primal yin and yang into life. We can see then if patients are using their resources appropriately to maintain health, well-being and achieve their purpose for being here. We can easily see if those resources are depleted and in need of postnatal support.

EMBRACING OUR DESTINY

In Figure 2.1 we can see the 8 EV configured in a way that shows the unfolding of jing and the development of the psyche. The 8 EV support the growth and development of not only the physical body but also the mental-emotional and spiritual growth that defines who we are. We can view the Chong Mai as the source of life and the birthplace of our curriculum in this configuration.

The Chong Mai receives the genetic material from previous generations but it can also be seen as the vessel through which the spirit determines to become earthbound in a physical body. The ability of the Chong Mai to link pre and postnatal qi through its influence on the kidneys, spleen and stomach allows for the transition from the "unity" or oneness of the source into a state of polarity that creates the potential for a postnatal experience.

So, it can be said that the undifferentiated yin and yang of the Chong Mai gives birth to Primal yin (Ren Mai) and Primal yang (Du Mai). This polarity or division of oneness gives us the ability to interact with the world around us. The Ren Mai provides us with the Yin or substances that source our postnatal journey. It gives us the building materials needed to have a life. The Du Mai provides the motive force to construct something with those resources. Then of course we may see the Chong Mai as the blueprint for the building of that life.

Since we do not live life in a static state, time becomes a factor in how we use the resources from this first ancestry (Chong, Ren and Du). The Wei vessels have the capacity to link the past with the future. They actively record life as we live it. They register our experiences and our responses to those experiences. In some ways, we can view these vessels as helping us to develop a coping style that helps us to deal with the ups and downs of life. They help us to determine how we might use the resources we have been given and how we use those resources determines how content we are with our life. If the Wei vessels are functioning in a healthy manner then we are able to learn from our experiences and embrace the new opportunities that we are given by life. If the vessels are overwhelmed or damaged by painful experiences then these vessels will try to keep us from moving on. They will keep us "stuck" in the past or longing for a future that can conquer the hurts of the past. A future that will make everything okay. We may be stuck in a fantasy or immobilized by the fear of future imagined pain and disappointment.

We live our childhoods in a state of dependency. We rely on our parents or caregivers to survive and thrive. We also rely on them to teach us values and how to succeed in life. It is from them that we learn what a successful life looks like. We take that knowledge when we leave the nest they have provided for us and we try to apply what we have learned. The process of individuation requires us to take what we have been taught by others and measure it against who we know ourselves to be. Do we have the same values as our parents, families or culture? In order to live our own lives we must at some point take a stand in who we are and how we will relate to the world around us. We must eventually make our own way. To do that, we must determine which of those values are resonant with who we are and which are not. We can love our parents, respect their values, appreciate their standards for a successful life and choose to live differently.

We must also align ourselves with some aspect of the world around us. Can we be present to who we are in this moment and then decide how we will participate in the world around us?

Will we make an effort to participate in the world in a way that is in alignment with who we are or will we live a life that is based on who others perceive us to be? That is the job of the Qiao vessels. They help us to use the resources of the first ancestry in the present moment to develop a healthy perspective on who we are and also on the world around us. They help us to take a stand here and now based on our perspective.

The Dai Mai is the last vessel in this process. The Dai Mai is the system's way of saying that no matter how bad or overwhelming life gets we will do whatever we need to in order to survive. Even the strongest of us may be overwhelmed by tragedy or trauma. How do we survive it? How do we manage in the face of insurmountable pain and continue to put one foot in front of the other? How do we keep going when our will to survive is fading away?

The 8 EV represent everything given to us to fulfill our destiny, including a way to survive the worst that life throws at us. The Dai Mai provides a container far away from the heart and the mind where we can store those events or emotions that overwhelm us and make us doubt our will to continue. The idea is that with time and perspective we will eventually be able to face that which we once pushed away. The memory of those experiences is repressed. It is stuffed down into the lower burner, far removed from the ever accessible memories in blood and captured in jing. They are far away from the consciousness of the heart/shen. If there are too many traumas or events that are unprocessed, the Dai Mai will use dampness to weigh things down and keep them contained. The containment then weighs down the spirit, taking the joy out of life leading to depression and apathy. If we are unable in our lifetimes to process these events then they are stored in the jing of the Chong Mai and passed on to the next generation.

In the development of the psyche, problems/pathology can occur anywhere in the process. One can be deprived of constitutional resources, which means we may have limited resources or diminished capacity with which to build. Life may have been harsh or cruel to us, damaging our desire to embrace future opportunities. We may have been overprotected or neglected by our primary caregivers early in life, affecting our ability to know and trust ourselves enough to be present in the moment and move out into the world. Or we may have been traumatized by life so significantly that we have forgotten who we are and our will to live or desire for experience is weighed down by the dampness we generate to forget.

So this configuration of the 8 EV gives us a map that guides us in a way that we are able to see what stage of development may be problematic in our patient's current state of distress.

CHAPTER 3

THE CHONG MAI

aka: The Thrusting Vessel, The Penetrating
Vessel, The Qi Thoroughfare

The Chong Mai can be seen as the source of all vessels. It is said to be undifferentiated yin and yang. It is the Sea of Blood (yin) and the Sea of Yuan Qi (yang). It is the Sea of the Five Zang Organs (yin) and the Sea of the Six Fu Organs (yang). This combination of yin and yang means that the Chong Mai contains within it all the resources necessary for life. It represents pure potential, unity and wholeness. This is the vessel that contains the genetic information from previous generations, passed on by the parents. It is the vessel responsible for the transmission of essence from one generation to the next. The wholeness or unity of the Chong Mai gives birth to yin and yang and that yin and yang is then manifested in a number of different expressions.

The Chong Mai is unique among the 8 EV. Its five branches cover a large area of the body from the tip of the toes to the top of the head. Its strong influence on the stomach and kidney channels provides a deep connection between prenatal and postnatal resources. It is a bridge between our prenatal experience in the womb and our new postnatal existence. It is also the bridge between us and the generations that have come before. You could say that the Chong Mai has the function of maintaining the continuity of a lineage. That continuity may give our lives meaning or it may be the ball and chain around our ankle that is creating impediments to our full expression of Self.

The prenatal function of the Chong Mai acts as a reservoir for the DNA (essence/jing) that is transmitted to us from our parents at the time of conception and during gestation. The Chong Mai is where the seed of our individual destiny is planted. This is the place from which our curriculum for life is sourced. It contains the essence of who we are and the potential for what we can become at the level of Yuan Shen (Original Spirit).

Once we are born, the Chong Mai creates the link between the prenatal and postnatal existence, connecting us to our lineage, our family history, and also creating a home for the most authentic aspect of who we are. This connection can be easily seen in the pathway of the Chong Mai and the points along the pathway. The master point of this vessel, Sp-4/Gong Sun Grandfather/Grandson, implies a link through the generations that goes beyond our parents, implying that our inheritance does not come from our parents alone. The gifts we manifest in this lifetime may come from many generations before us.

The Chong Mai has a significant number of points from the Kidney, Spleen and Stomach channels further supporting its capacity to link prenatal (Kidney) and postnatal qi (Spleen and Stomach). The Kidney points are predominantly located on the trunk (Ki-12 through Ki-27) and the Spleen and Stomach points can be found on the legs beginning with St-30 where the legs attach to the trunk and continuing down to the toes (see Figure 3.1). It is interesting to me that the prenatal aspect (Kidney) is close to the core of who we are (trunk) and the postnatal function (Spleen and Stomach) directs each step (legs) we take along the journey. The prenatal aspect contains within it all the resources we have been given for our journey and the postnatal aspect of the Chong Mai are the steps we take to disseminate, feed and support those resources.

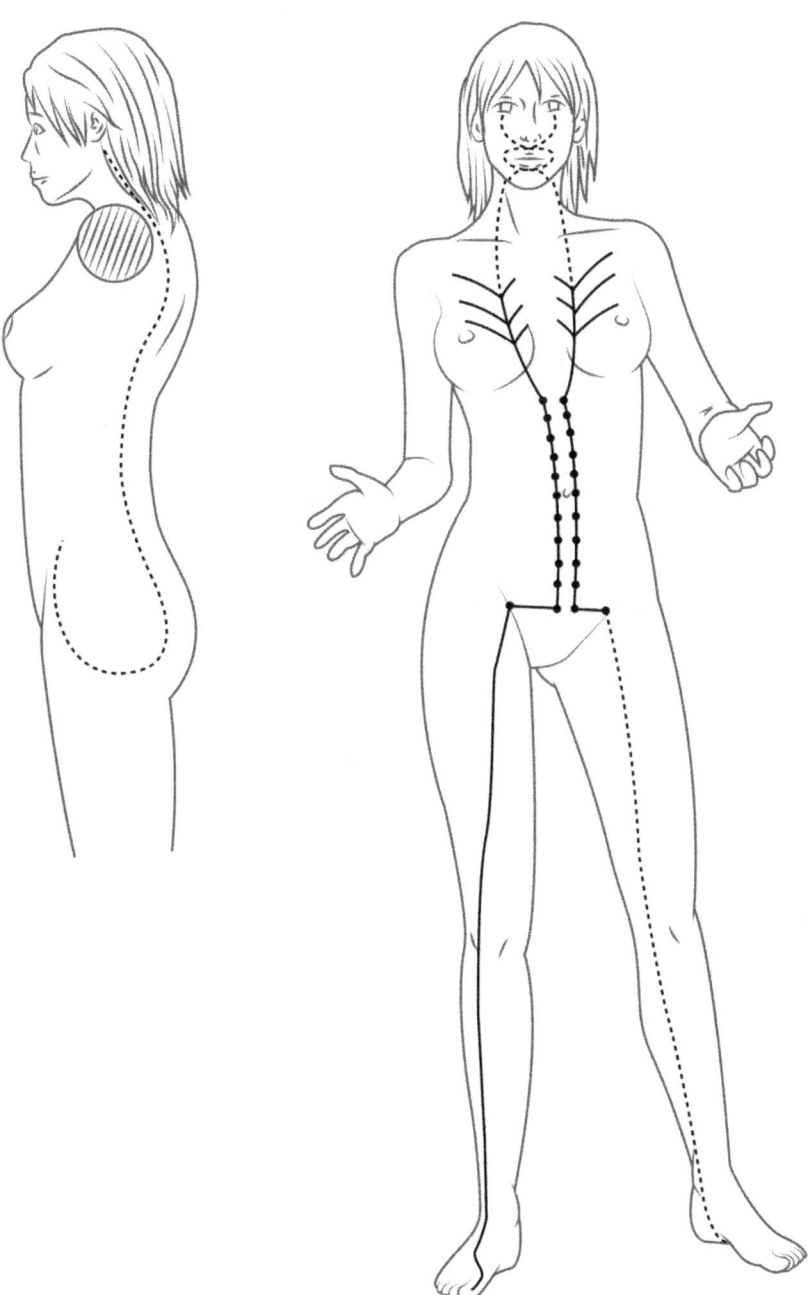

Figure 3.1: Chong Mai

CHONG MAI AND CREATION

In some creation myths G-d creates the Universe/World by contracting in on Itself making a space for additional aspects of the G-d-self to come into being. G-d creates an act of separation by contracting deep within Itself allowing for the opportunity and space for something else to exist. You can see this in the cell division of a fertilized ovum—this single cell that contains all it needs, all that is passed down through time. In the act of cell division/creation it contracts in on itself and then divides. First into two cells, then those cells contract and become four and the four become eight and the eight become the many.

This act of creation can be seen as a selfless act, an act of boredom or even an act of curiosity. Whatever your perspective, it seems reasonable to then infer that for experience to exist, first the one must become two (yin and yang) and the two become the many. Since the Chong Mai is "the one" or "the all" of prenatal existence, it follows that in order for us to have a postnatal experience or a human experience, the Chong Mai must give birth to the polarity of Primal Yin (Ren Mai) and Primal Yang (Du Mai) and from this first act of separation/creation, the two become the many.

This act of creation is a powerful one but also one that comes at a cost to the spirit. The spirit experiences this act of creation as a separation from the whole. It is a break, if you will, and therefore there will be an instinctual drive to repair the break or return to the whole. The prenatal aspect of the Chong Mai is unity and the postnatal expression is forever trying to return to that unity.

If we grow up in an environment that is filled with love and we are reminded often that we are indeed valuable and perfect just the way we are, then perhaps that drive to repair is less demanding or it doesn't force itself into action until later in life when disappointment or failure raise their heads. But the drive to repair or return to unity will eventually assert itself. This is especially true if our early childhood has been less than idyllic and we have from a very early age felt as if we are broken. When the drive or urge to return happens we start to ask ourselves those existential questions:

- "Who am I?"

- "Why am I here?"

- "What is my purpose?"

- "What is the meaning of life?"

- "Is this all there is?"

- "What does it mean to be whole?"

The strength of the Chong Mai is in its ability to remind us that we have everything that we need to journey through life. It reminds us who we are at the core. It is the source of our authenticity. It is the vessel that can offer up the clearest, most true version of our being-ness. It gives us access to that part of who we are that is perfect, unbroken and capable of anything. Remembering that part of ourselves can remind us that we are spiritual beings having an earthly experience and that experience cannot change the quality and the content of our light.

The Chong Mai also connects us to our lineages (blood and spirit). In receiving the Heavenly Mandate through the procreative act we become part of a spiritual lineage just like we become part of the familial and cultural lineages through our parents. Because the Chong Mai comes from the contributions of essence/jing given to us by our parents we are expected to take the good with the bad. If our parents cannot supply healthy essence or sufficient essence then we are left to deal with the deficit as part of our curriculum. We are left to find a postnatal way of existing that not only makes the best use of what we have been given but also finds ways of living that support the deficit. Let's say you were born into a big family. If you were lucky to be first in line and your mom and dad were in their early 20s then you can celebrate the fact that you likely received the best essence/jing that your parents had to offer. If on the other hand you were the tenth in line and your mom was in her 40s and she had trouble conceiving and carrying you and two of your previously born siblings, you may have to deal with the fact that you were a little short-sheeted in the essence department. For those of you who have never been short-sheeted or do not understand that term, I highly recommend Googling it. This means that you may have to deal with the fact that your prenatal resources may be less than optimal and you may need to support them with postnatal resources. So you may be less able to ignore the communication from your body or you may pay a bigger price for ignoring those needs. You may be more vulnerable to certain diseases or emotional imbalances. You may tire more easily than your siblings, you may be more easily overwhelmed or you may have less drive or ambition. This does not mean that *you* are less than. It only means that your diminished resources become part of your curriculum and the sooner you recognize and accept that, the sooner you will be able to use those resources in the most effective manner.

Another way you might see this is in your immune system. If you were born with a weakness in your constitution that makes you vulnerable to illness then you must make lifestyle and dietary choices that can help you to overcome or at the very least be less vulnerable to disease. If your family lineage includes a lot of cancer, that vulnerability or predisposition is passed down through the Chong Mai and you must then use the postnatal Chong Mai to support a healthy lifestyle including not only diet and exercise but also how you deal with stress. In addition, you would be also wise to consider what limiting beliefs you might have about the inevitability that you too will someday have cancer. Although you have been given the imprint or genetic predisposition for this disease you have also been gifted with the free will that may be the defining element in whether or not that predisposition is ever expressed. This is the difference between genetics and epigenetics. We might consider that the Chong Mai can be used to help the patient alter gene expression.

CHONG MAI AND INTERGENERATIONAL TRAUMA

Traumatic experience may also be transmitted from one generation to the next. This may help to explain why certain types of mental illness run in families. Unresolved or overwhelming traumas are stored in the bones of the traumatized person. This means that the imprint of those traumas ends up in our jing and that jing is then transmitted to the next generation. We may be carrying the wounds of our parents and their parents before them. Some traumas are passed down for many generations. This may manifest itself in feelings of fear, anxiety, guilt, shame and lack of self-esteem that may appear to be unfounded or unjustifiable based on our present circumstances. We may be living with feelings of being "less than" that have more to do with something that happened to our great-great-grandparents than anything that currently exists in our lives.

I often think of the generations that have followed those who survived the Holocaust. The overwhelming physical and emotional trauma of that time must have left a powerful imprint on the essence of the survivors. How could one possibly survive the deprivation, torture and fear of that time without some lingering impact on their jing. Trauma like that not only marks the soul, it also changes the DNA.

Here's the good news: as the trauma is passed down to the next generation, so is the strength that comes from maintaining one's humanity in the face of the trauma. The Chong Mai is the vehicle for this transmission. I imagine that African-Americans who come from enslaved ancestors carry that trauma in their DNA. They must also carry the resilience and strength of those who survived in the face of unimaginable trauma. The question then becomes what do you feed, the trauma or the resilience? Do you focus on the deficit or do you know that you can, because of that lineage, rise like a phoenix from the ashes? Surviving, empowered by the resilience and the ability to overcome against all odds. If you can accept that you have received this imprint then you can use your free will to rise above it. Even more importantly, with consciousness and effort you can break the chain for future generations.

Those are big, easily accessible examples of trans-generational trauma but there is evidence of it everywhere. Family histories of depression, addiction and anxiety all have some basis in this idea of trans-generational trauma. I have treated many patients who suffer from anxiety and/or depression who feel as if they are living with a family legacy. Their parents or grandparents also suffered. They fear, because it was passed down from one generation to the next, that they have no way of overcoming it, as if it is a done deal. It might be very healing to know when this began in their family history. Was there a precipitating event? Was there war or famine or an epidemic that stirred this emotional response that was unresolved and then passed down? Treating the Chong Mai can free us from the weight of this transmission and may actually even break the chain for future generations. If we do the work of the Chong Mai we may be able to prevent the next generations from carrying the burden of trauma from the previous generations.

CHONG MAI AND CULTURAL EXPECTATION

With this link to our lineage the Chong Mai also governs our relationship to cultural or familial expectations. My grandfather was an engineer, my father was an engineer and like it or not there was some expectation in our family that one of my siblings or I would be an engineer. So, thankfully for the world of engineering, it was not me. Although, I can honestly say that some days I think like an engineer and I do have a fondness for flow charts. Good with the bad.

This cultural or familial expectation can be very deeply rooted and the source of much suffering for individuals who love their parents and their culture but have very different ideas about how they want to live their lives. I once treated a patient who suffered from intense feelings of guilt and anxiety because she did not want to fulfill her familial obligations to return to her home and marry the person her parents would choose. These feelings prevented her from fully expressing who she was and they also made having a significant relationship of her choosing very challenging.

THE FIVE TRAJECTORIES OF THE CHONG MAI

Each of the five trajectories has its own unique contribution to the functions of the Chong Mai. Three of the trajectories are ascending in nature and two are descending in nature. I like to think of the ascending pathways as the way we bring that prenatal jing to shen, linking the blood to essence and bringing the functions of thinking and feeling into consciousness. The descending branches ground us into the earth, aiding the postnatal function of the spleen and stomach. These descending branches create an anchor for the spiritual ascension of the Chong Mai. They support our postnatal processing system. It is common when treating the Chong Mai to use one or two branches only in any given treatment.

First trajectory

Points: Ren-2, Ki-11, St-30, Sp-12, Ki-12 through Ki-21

This is the primary pathway of the Chong Mai. It connects the heart and the uterus (upper and lower mansions of blood). It originates in the lower jiao (uterus in women) and descends to the pubic bone where it emerges and spreads to St-30 and Sp-12. Here it returns to the midline and ascends the center of the body (along the kidney channel) to end at the diaphragm and spread in the chest.

In this trajectory we see issues related to the inability to link prenatal and postnatal qi. This most often manifests as Kidney yang failing to support Spleen qi.

Birth trauma, serious illness or dietary issues in the first cycle of jing can be the underlying etiology for pathology in this branch. One might see this as illness or suffering from the moment an infant crosses from a prenatal to postnatal existence. Infants may suffer from a failure to thrive or as they grow they may fail to meet typical developmental markers.

In adults we typically see a long history, often from birth or early childhood, of people who have difficulty digesting life. This may stem from not having their physiological or emotional needs met. Children spend much of their first cycle of jing developing and building their postnatal function. If their prenatal qi is strong there is support for that development. If, however, there is birth trauma then this impedes the transition between pre and postnatal qi. If, after birth, the infant's nutritional needs are not met through difficulties with lactation or trouble digesting premade formulas then the capacity to build postnatal qi is compromised. When the process of weaning is challenging, or if the child develops food sensitivities or allergies with the introduction of solid foods, that frequently presents later in life with a weakness in the function of Earth (Spleen and Stomach).

Adults with this pathology may present with a multitude of digestive problems including:

- assimilation disorders

- chronic diarrhea or constipation

- food retention

- food allergies

- food intolerances like lactose intolerance

- celiac disease

- leaky gut syndrome.

These patients may also display an inability to digest life from an emotional perspective. They may suffer from emotional eating, chronic fatigue, chronic depression or an inability to pursue new ideas or bring context to current experiences. These patients often are like hamsters running on a wheel. They are exhausted but they keep on running because they cannot think clearly enough to get off the wheel. Their ability to transform and transport is compromised, which means they do not have enough yuan qi to change.

Second trajectory

Points: Ki-22 through Ki-27, Ren-22, Ren-23, St-1

This pathway is often thought of as the Ren Mai trajectory. This pathway allows for jing to connect to all of the other fluids/humors in the region of the chest and face. In this pathway, the postnatal function of the stomach as the "origin of fluids" supplies the clear fluids that are then ascended to the chest and follow the pathway of the Ren Mai around the mouth and up to the eyes at St-1. It allows for blood and fluids to be brought to the face, nourishing the sensory orifices. This pathway is responsible for clarity in the sensory orifices. If one lacks the capacity to send blood and clear fluids up to the head to nourish the sensory orifices then our capacity to receive information through those portals may be impaired. We may be prone to dizziness or light-headedness or we may have difficulty with perception based on lack of clarity affecting how information from the world outside gets in.

The link to the chest connects the greater luo-collaterals of the spleen (Sp-21), stomach (Xu Li/Empty Mile) and Ren Mai (Ren-15) together allowing for the management of blood flow in the chest. The kidney shu points on the chest (Ki-22 through Ki-27) gather and mediate the yin resources (humors) of jing, blood and body fluids.

Each of the five kidney shu points from Ki-22 to Ki-26 have both a five element association and a connection to the shen through the five spirits and Ki-27 is the master shu creating harmony or balance in the other five.

Ki-26	Metal	Po Corporeal Soul
Ki-25	Fire	Shen Spirit/Mind
Ki-24	Wood	Hun Ethereal Soul
Ki-23	Earth	Yi Thought
Ki-22	Water	Zhi Will

Obstruction in this branch leads to blood stasis in the chest and rebellious qi, resulting in:

- anxiety and panic attacks

- running piglet/internal urgency

- vomiting

- chest pain.

These patients may have forgotten who they are. They have lost the connection to their heart. Their spirits lack nourishment and so they lose that deep sense of self that encourages them to live from the place of "everything I need is available to me."

The second trajectory also reinforces the connection between the heart and kidney. When this connection is intact people are able to find meaning in their experiences. When the Chong Mai maintains the relationship between the heart and kidney, whatever challenges, traumas or illnesses we experience may be understood in a way that helps us to grow and become more of who we are. It brings our curriculum (jing) into the light of shen so that our journey will have meaning and purpose. It is at this level that patients are able to clearly pursue their destiny with heart instead of losing will and laying down to fate. If we lack this connection we lose the meaning and purpose and we are prone to pursuing passions and desires that do not serve our growth. We are reckless in our desires and unsatisfied when we fulfill them. We accomplish something and then feel emptiness in the face of that accomplishment because whatever it was we thought we wanted was not based in the healthy relationship between the heart and the kidneys, essence and blood. It lacked meaning and ultimately it had nothing to do with our purpose for being here.

Third trajectory
Points: Ren-2, St-30, GB-26, Du-1 (Du-4), UB-17

As I mentioned earlier, the Chong Mai is the source vessel that gives birth to primal yin and primal yang. In the second branch we see the expression of primal yin and in the third branch we see the connection to primal yang. The Chong Mai engages the motive force of yang and uses that force to propel blood and hold everything in place. The Chong uses the pathway of the Dai Mai (originating from Du-4 to encircle the waist) to access the Du Mai. This branch has an impact on cognition and memory. It does this by insuring that blood flows to the brain and the heart and by supporting the Du Mai function of governing the Sea of Marrow (brain and spinal cord). There is a sense of vitality that may fade if this branch is impeded. When patients lose the fire of Ming Men and the motive force of yang we can see the loss of will, apathy and the capacity for clear thinking. The memory is affected because the Sea of Blood fails to nourish the brain and heart. Conditions like senile dementia, amnesia or aphasia associated with loss of cognitive function can be seen here. Physiologically one might see pain from blood stasis affecting the lower jiao, joints and spine. We might also see the loss of yang resulting in qi sinking or damp accumulation from a lack of fire for transformation and transportation. The loss of the motive force of yang that comes from the Du Mai branch means that we simply don't care about our purpose for being here. What drive we had to pursue meaning in life, to pursue the destiny given to us by the resources of the Chong Mai is waning like a pilot light in an old furnace. It just isn't strong enough to ignite the flames to heat the air that warms the house. Or, in the words of the mighty king of blues, B.B. King, "The thrill is gone."

Fourth trajectory

Points: Ki-11, Ki-10, UB-40, Ki-6 through Ki-3, Kidney Prime

The fourth trajectory travels downward into the legs from the groin and has a strong connection to the Qiao vessels. This branch helps people feel connected to the earth and allows them to move with ease. It brings jing to the bones in the feet. It supports posture, because the alignment of posture begins in the feet. It also brings yang to the spleen.

Imbalances in this branch can be seen to affect a child when they begin to walk. It may cause the first steps to be either too early or too late. If it forces the energy for walking to emerge too early there may be a deficit in neurological function as the brain has not had sufficient time developing through sitting and crawling. If the walking begins too late other forms of development may also be delayed. We may also see struggles in learning to walk later as the increased body weight may make it harder to find the balance and strength to support that weight. Health in this pathway means that walking begins when the structure is ready to support the body weight. Since walking upright is also related to the Du Mai, the discussion about how this unfolds in a child will continue in Chapter 5.

In adults we may see postural problems especially related to a weakness in the legs and poor contact with the ground. This may also show up as an instability in the mental-emotional process. For the mental-emotional process to be stable, one must be grounded. Stability or grounding comes in three forms through the Chong Mai. The first is the relationship to the kidneys. This branch of the Chong Mai travels to the bottom of the foot to Kidney Prime and therefore represents the grounding that comes from feeling your feet contacting the ground. The second way the Chong Mai supports grounding is through the earth (spleen and stomach) and the third is through the blood. The earth provides stability by governing movement in the center of the body. The more stable the middle is the more stable the emotional life is. When the middle is obstructed or too weak, the ability to process experience is compromised and the ability to remain calm and think our way through things is affected. As for the blood, the stability that the blood provides is like the ballast on a boat. It is a dense form of yin that provides the material basis for the mind. So when the blood is sufficient and circulating it provides a stability that is like the weights (ballast) that boat makers use to keep boats upright and stable in stormy seas. The descending or grounding nature of this branch can also treat asthma and some digestive problems by redirecting the qi flow downward and restoring stability.

Fifth trajectory
Points: St-30, St-36, St-37, St-39, St-42, Lv-1, Sp-1

The pathway of the fifth trajectory supports the relationship between the spleen qi and liver blood. The lower he-sea points of the Stomach, Large Intestine and Small Intestine (St-36, St-37, St-39) are on this pathway so it can easily be said that this branch affects how we assimilate and also how we separate clear from turbid. This branch impacts the spleen's function of transformation and transportation. When the spleen is functioning well it initiates the generation of blood, which is stored by the liver. If the spleen qi and liver blood are sufficient they will support the kidney yin.

Are we digesting life in a way that supports our curriculum? This branch can help to support the healthy lifestyle choices that are necessary to maintain and conserve our prenatal resources. It is useful in generating enough postnatal resources (qi and blood) to avoid having to deplete the prenatal resources (kidney yin) we were gifted for our journey.

Patients who benefit from the treatment of this branch typically have a wide range of digestive disorders but also in some way are having difficulty digesting life. Their physical complaints are exacerbated by emotional stress. When patients are under pressure or feeling overwhelmed the liver qi stagnates, impeding the spleen's ability to function appropriately. As a descending pathway sometimes you see patients "lose their footing" when life becomes too much for them. They cannot generate sufficient blood for ballast so they are easy to knock over from an emotional point of view. I find this branch affected frequently in patients who want me to tell them where to go and what to do. They are not grounded enough to make their own decisions and having someone else decide for them creates a sense of stability and decreases stress levels—assuming, that is, you can trust the person making the decisions.

Ultimately, the Chong Mai is the bridge between prenatal and postnatal qi. It is the source of all the other vessels and the place where our core being-ness resides. It links us to our lineage, which in some ways is anchoring and supporting and in another is a repository of generational baggage that is there for us to work through. Regardless, it is the place where we can remember who we are…spirit, light, love, perfection.

PHYSIOLOGICAL IMPACT OF THE CHONG MAI

While we are learning to recognize the archetypal nature of this vessel and how imbalance in the Chong Mai can create suffering of a certain nature, we can always rely on the physical manifestations to help us make our diagnosis. There are a number of common conditions that are consistent with Chong Mai pathology and because we know the body and mind are one, if there is a problem in our curriculum associated with the Chong Mai there will be some physical manifestation of that pathology.

Common conditions treated by the Chong Mai

- Gynecological problems associated with blood deficiency, blood stasis, blood heat and kidney deficiency.

- Any condition that affects the Three Treasures (Jing, Qi and Shen), Kidneys, Spleen and Stomach, and Heart.

- Qi counterflow: Hot face with cold feet, fullness and distention in the trunk, internal urgency, running piglet.

- Lumps in the throat or breast (plum-pit, thyroid issues, cystic breasts).

- Insufficient hair growth: beard in men, head hair for women. Also excessive facial hair in women (often associated with Poly Cystic Ovarian Syndrome (PCOS)).

- "Nine Kinds of Heart Pain": arrhythmias, anxiety and palpitations.

- Morning sickness or any stomach excess syndrome.

- Asthma due to rebellious qi or phlegm stagnation.

- Atrophy of the legs.

CHAPTER 4

THE REN MAI

aka: The Conception Vessel, The Directing Vessel,
The Sea of Yin, The Sea of Containment,
The Vessel of Closure and The Channel of Bonding

This vessel is the primary reservoir of yin. To understand the Ren Mai one must therefore understand the nature of yin. A simple way to understand yin is to compare it to the nature of yang.

Yin	Yang
Dark	Light
Wet	Dry
Cool	Warm
Contractive	Expansive
Soft	Hard
Quiescent	Active
Substance	Function
Containment	Expression

An imbalance in the Ren Mai can result in yin excess, yin stasis or yin deficiency. Over-nourishment results in yin excess (phlegm, damp and yin stasis) and under-nourishment of the Ren Mai can result in yin deficiency.

Another way to understand the Ren Mai is to look at its archetypal nature. This vessel represents the archetype of the Feminine, especially the archetype of the Mother. It is no accident that this vessel's name is most often translated as the Conception vessel. There is a strong relationship between the Ren Mai and gestation, labor, birth and mothering processes. This archetypal energy may be active in anyone, male or female, mother, father or someone who does not have children at all, because the vessel itself is about the capacity to conceive of something, hold and nourish that thing (gestation), give birth to it and support its growth. This may be a business, a garden, a work of art, four-legged children (pets) or even someone else's children. It is about our capacity to love and nourish in way that fully expresses who we are.

The energy of the Mother is vital to how we navigate the world. The Ren Mai is the vessel that infuses us with self-love and insures that we have the resources we need to make our way in the world. If a mother is unable to bond with her infant for any number of reasons, including post-partum depression, addiction or even a poor relationship with her own mother then the baby may suffer. The loss of yin resources means that babies and then the adults they become often feel under-nourished, abandoned or unworthy of love.

When we speak of this we are speaking of the actual mother but the truth is, the Ren Mai is an energy that can be supplied by anyone. So if another individual steps in and supplies the necessary bonding and yin then the baby has a better chance of developing in a healthy manner.

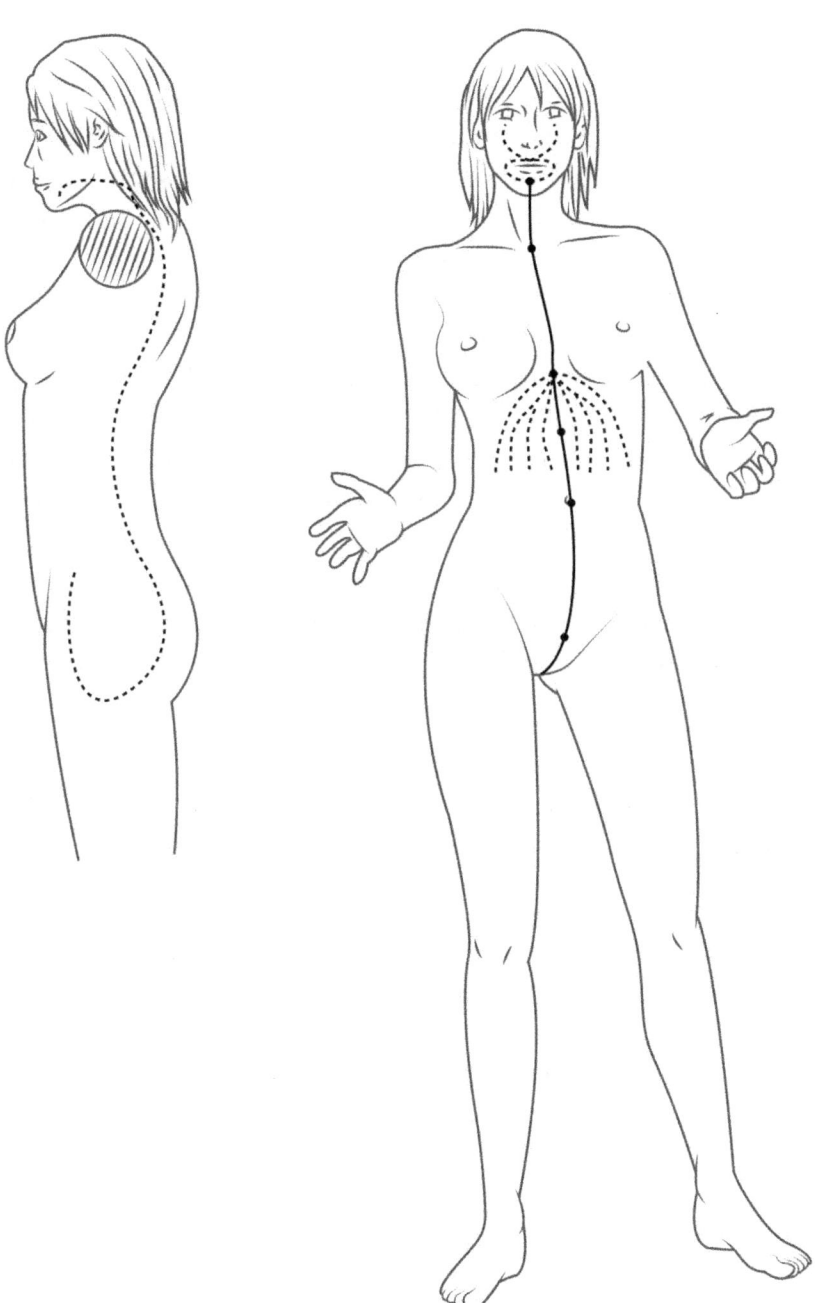

Figure 4.1: Ren Mai

REN MAI AND BIRTH TRAUMA

When we are born the process is a traumatic one. We are forced by uterine contractions into the birth canal and with time and great effort we enter the world. If we are lucky, someone has taken care in making that transition as minimally traumatic as possible. But even if we are lucky, birth is still a shock. We arrive from a place that is dark, warm and muffles sound into a dramatic/traumatic increase in sensory input. We come into the light of the room and our senses are no longer buffered by the darkness of the womb and the amniotic fluids (yin). Then we have to transition from an oxygen-rich environment supplied to us by blood (more yin) into fighting for our own breath (yang). Our lungs inflating as we struggle with our new-found need to bring the outside world in. Finally, someone cuts the cord that is our connection to our source of nourishment and now we must seek nourishment outside of the safety of the womb.

Even under the best of circumstances we are distressed. Imagine how much worse that trauma might be if a baby had to suffer a premature delivery, a forceps delivery or perhaps suffered shoulder dystocia. Or imagine what it would be like to suffer those original three traumas of birth through a C-section that causes the shock of sudden decompression when the uterine wall is quickly opened.

Part of the Ren Mai function is to heal the traumas of birth, like how a mother's hug makes everything all better. In a conscious birthing process the newly born infant is placed immediately on the mother's bare chest. The baby's Ren Mai (cheek) is connected to the mother's Ren Mai. This connection Ren to Ren and the sound of the mother's heartbeat and respiration help the baby to make the transition from a prenatal to a postnatal existence. The healing continues as the mother nurses and bonds with the baby. These acts are a large part of what helps a child to feel loved and supported, which allows for closure on the traumas of birth.

In utero we have no sense of separateness from the mother and once thrust into the world we feel the loss of connection and we are driven by nature to find union. When babies breastfeed it is an opportunity to reconnect with the familiar. The suckling connects the Ren of the mother and child. Infants automatically synchronize their breathing and heartbeat with their mother's. They gaze into the mother's eyes affirming their existence and value. They feel loved. All of these acts connect us to the source of primal yin.

If at any time during this process the mother is overly stressed, anxious or depressed, the bonding process is impaired. This bonding is essential to a child's sense of self and to their ability to exist in the world with a sense of security.

So it is interesting to consider how many of us actually have this optimal birth transition. How many women give birth in environments that respect the sanctity of birth and recognize the need to make it less traumatic? In the US attitudes towards birth and the period of time right after birth are improving but they are nowhere near optimal. This leads to increased stress in mothers, which hinders the ability to bond appropriately.

Insufficient bonding in the first cycle of jing (seven years for girls, eight years for boys) may lead to an inability of the individual to bond in adulthood. This is especially true in the first two years. This in turn makes relationships very challenging. For, truly, if we cannot love ourselves how can we love another? If we feel that we are not worthy of the basic yin resources in life because those things were not available to us in our first few years of life then we may try to manipulate others in order to get what we need. We may feel that we have to earn our right to exist. We may care for others only because we hope they will in turn care for us. If we do not get the chance to experience unconditional love early in life, how can we be expected to feel it for another?

REN MAI AND SELF-CARE

Insufficient self-care is a very typical issue in those who have Ren Mai imbalances. Caretakers who deny themselves what they need in order to care for others are common Ren Mai patterns. Patients who have this imbalance do not appreciate that if they do not care for themselves then they will be unable to continue caring for others. For these patients, I often use the airplane metaphor, reminding them that in the case of an emergency, flight attendants instruct people travelling with children to put the oxygen mask on themselves FIRST before placing the mask on their child.

REN MAI AND NOURISHMENT

Eating disorders or unhealthy relationships with food are also often based in Ren Mai imbalances. People often turn to food for comfort when they are deprived of other resources. They often learn this at the hands of the well-meaning caregivers. If you fall down and hurt yourself a cookie will make everything feel better. This need to distract from discomfort or fill the feelings of pain, emptiness or aloneness with food creates a pathological bond to food that may lead to eating disorders or obesity.

If the Ren Mai is healthy in infancy and babies are loved and supported in an appropriate fashion then children can learn to self-soothe. If the opposite is true then the ability to self-soothe may never be developed and individuals will turn to food or other substances to numb out the overwhelming feelings or anxiety produced by living in a world of lack.

So the energy of the Ren Mai is essential in healthy bonding and the ability to connect with self and others in a way that is nourishing and loving.

REN MAI AND CLOSURE

One of the other gifts of the Ren Mai is the ability to create closure or let go. This is actually part of the self-care process. If we care enough for ourselves then we can let go of the experiences or people in our lives that no longer serve us or support us. Another way this supports us is our capacity to surrender to what is so that we can make room for that which will serve us. In other words, an inability to let go of the past or accept the present impedes our ability to create or receive a future that is in alignment with our purpose.

REN MAI AND QI STAGNATION

One of the other names of the Ren Mai is the Directing vessel. When qi is stagnant or rebelling the Ren Mai can encourage movement and redirect the qi flow. This is not unlike our mother's job as our first teacher. Our mothers encourage us to keep trying when we are learning new things or perhaps they redirect our efforts when we are frustrated or stuck. When we experience this type of support early in life we learn better how to deal with frustration, stress and failure.

Sometimes in childhood the Ren Mai is in excess. This may manifest in the form of the mother who is over-controlling or over-attached. When this happens, what we typically see is the qi stops moving effectively and yin starts to accumulate.

This excess yin may be in response to an inability to bond or self-soothe. If we are fearful or anxious sometimes the additional yin provides an artificial ballast that makes us feel calmer and more substantial. This can occur if we have fearful mothers who cannot contain their fear. Sometimes we are over-controlled early in life by mothers who suppress our movement into yang. These mothers limit a child's natural curiosity. They, in an effort to protect, thwart movement that seems too risky. This control leads to an accumulation of yin by blocking the movement of yang. So, if our primary caregivers do not know when to let us direct ourselves and become more independent then our qi becomes blocked, frustration occurs and yin accumulates.

REN MAI AND ADDICTION

Addiction is seen in CM as a loss of sovereignty of the heart. This is evidence, in part, of an inability to make connections and bond in a healthy manner. Opioids are naturally occurring reward brain chemicals. Infants depend on these naturally produced brain chemicals in their parents. So in a way we can say that endorphin highs are one of the ways that parents are rewarded for the efforts to love and care for their child. They are the essential component in the emotional apparatus in the brain responsible for protecting and nurturing. So especially in opiate addiction, what we see is that the mechanism of addiction occurs in a system that governs how we attach or bond. Addiction is a process that results from a naturally occurring but overwhelming drive to bond and feel love. Children who have not received appropriate or sufficient bonding may be more prone to seek a chemical substitution later in life.

Healthy bonding, which is dependent on the Ren Mai, creates a sense of connectedness in a child.

Recent research shows that if people are unable to bond, if they are isolated or unable to feel a part of a community, they will be more vulnerable to addiction.

The light in a mother's eyes, including the size of her pupils when she gazes at her child, has an *immediate* effect on a child's brain chemistry. If a child sees deep love and profound connection in their mother's eyes they will feel that they belong. The more they see that look, the more the brain aligns itself with a feeling in the child that they are enough. When these children become adults they are significantly less likely to need the endorphins produced by addictive substances or behaviors. Even if they become addicted through circumstance they will more likely overcome the addiction. The power of the Ren Mai is the power of love. It is the power of belonging.

REN MAI PATHWAY

The primary pathway of the Ren Mai originates in the lower abdomen (uterus in females), emerges in the perineum at Ren-1 and follows up the anterior midline of the trunk to Ren-24 where it encircles the mouth to connect with the Du Mai and then engages the stomach channel at St-4, 3, 2 and St-1. This connection to the stomach channel on the face explains some of the functions of the Ren Mai. The ability to maintain a healthy yin supply to the sensory orifices means we get to perceive the world in a healthy and more grounded way. It also reinforces the digestive aspect of the Ren Mai. Since digestion begins in the mouth, the connection to the stomach channel means we can have clarity about how we can best nourish ourselves. The Ren Mai connection to the stomach channel is also important when it comes to the generation of fluids. The Ren Mai is the source of prenatal fluids (Yin) and the stomach is the origin of postnatal fluids created in the process of digestion.

The Ren Mai also has a Du Mai branch, which reminds us of the inter-relationship between yin and yang. This branch originates in the lower abdomen and instead of moving towards the front of the body it turns towards the back of the body and ascends the spine. This connection to yang supports the Ren Mai ability to direct qi downward and influence the function of qi. It also maintains some of the interdependence between yin and yang.

Common conditions treated by the Ren Mai

- Gynecological issues associated with the seven/eight cycles of jing: menarche, puberty, infertility, menstrual irregularities, premenstrual syndrome, pregnancy, childbirth, post-partum and menopause.

- Dysfunction in the lower burner: genital conditions both male and female, constipation, diarrhea, urinary dysfunction and menstrual diseases, especially those related to qi stagnation or kidney deficiency.

- Fluid metabolism disorders—both excess and deficiency of fluids.

- Asthma due to Lung qi deficiency or Kidney failing to grasp qi.

- Yin deficiency conditions: Kidney yin deficiency affecting the Heart, Lungs, Liver and Stomach.

- Qi stagnation affecting all three burners.

- Masses in the lower burner due to qi stagnation: Shan disorders in men and gynecological masses in women.

CHAPTER 5

THE DU MAI

aka: The Governing Vessel, The Sea of
Individuation, The Vessel of Separation

The Du Mai is the Sea of Yang. It is the reservoir of primary
yang and it supplies the yang energy for motive force in the
world. It governs the yang organs and yang channels and can be
used to dispel yang pathogens such as heat and wind.

DU MAI AND INDEPENDENCE

At about the time a child begins to stand upright and walk the
Du Mai begins to assert itself. As the governing vessel or the
Sea of Individuation it gives the child the impulse to "separate"
from the maternal matrix. At this early stage of emergence of
yang, children cautiously begin to extend themselves out into
the world. They move away from their mothers and begin to
explore the world around them. Early in this process there
are frequent returns to the mother for comfort and a sense of
safety but eventually the child becomes braver with an increased
confidence in its ability to move in the world. Fathers or
caregivers (grandfathers, older siblings, uncles) can play a vital
role at this stage encouraging and modeling how to be more
adventuresome and courageous in their explorations. This is not
necessarily gender specific. A female family member can also
instill this courageousness in a child. It is not about gender; it's

about the ability to model healthy yang behavior. Eventually, with support and positive experiences, the periods of separation increase in time and distance. With every successful exploration the child becomes more willing to step away from the safety of the mother into an experience of their own.

Although we speak of nursing as being a Ren Mai issue because of the bonding that occurs, the Du Mai also has its part in the process. The activation of Du-14 Da Zhui, just below the seventh cervical vertebrae, provides the motive force to lift the head to allow the baby to see the breast and latch on. The lifting of the head becomes stronger over time and the baby begins to see the world around them. Eventually infants become toddlers. They gain in strength and the curiosity to explore that which they can see.

DU MAI AND MASTERY OF SPACE

The energy of Du-4 Ming Men provides the impulse to stand upright and investigate what the baby has seen. Over time as the Du Mai asserts itself there is a mastery of the space around them. The child begins to conquer the world, at first in small ways. They navigate around furniture, through doorways and up and down stairways. I once spent an hour with an 18-month-old child going up and down stairs. It was fascinating to watch this little girl negotiate her ability to step up and down. She even used the words "up" and "down" to lock in the experience. She did not want to stop this exercise until she felt a sense of mastery. She conquered those stairs and I had the backache to prove it.

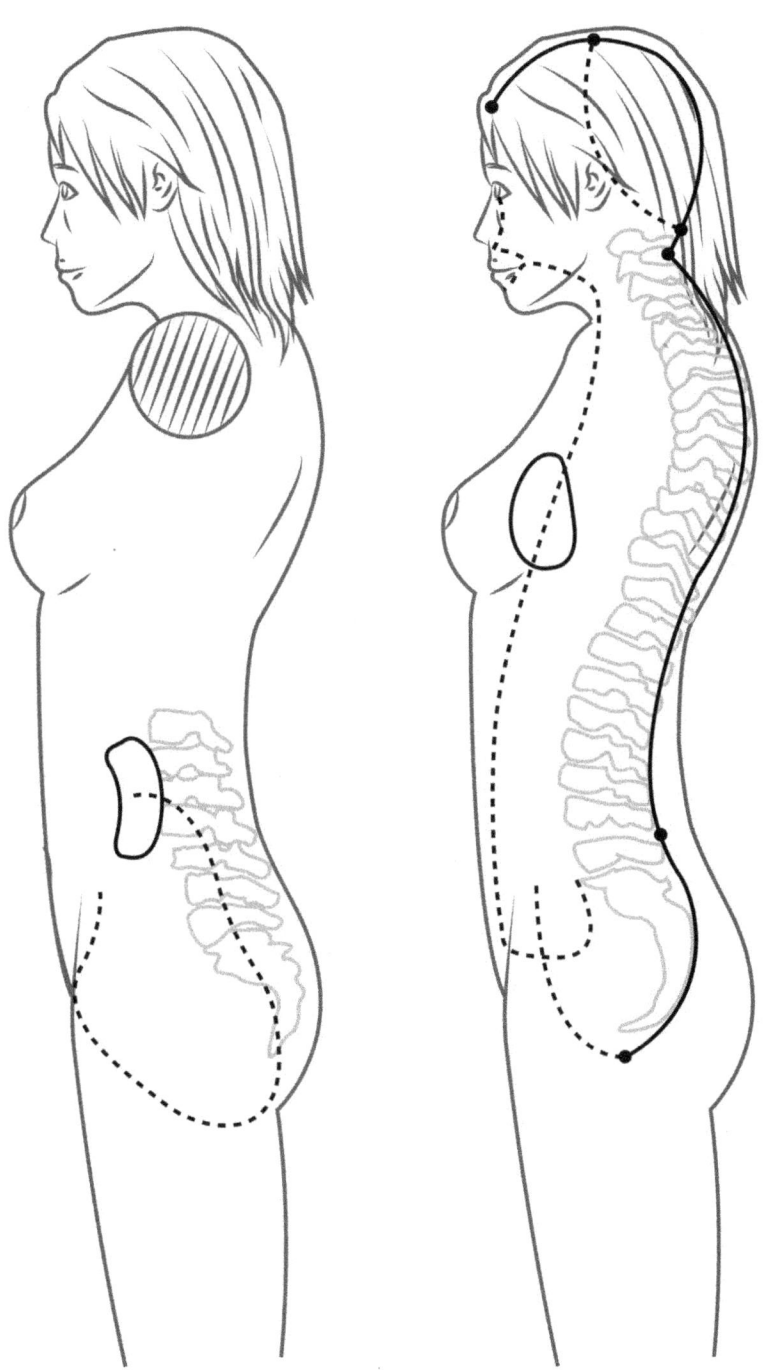

Figure 5.1: Du Mai

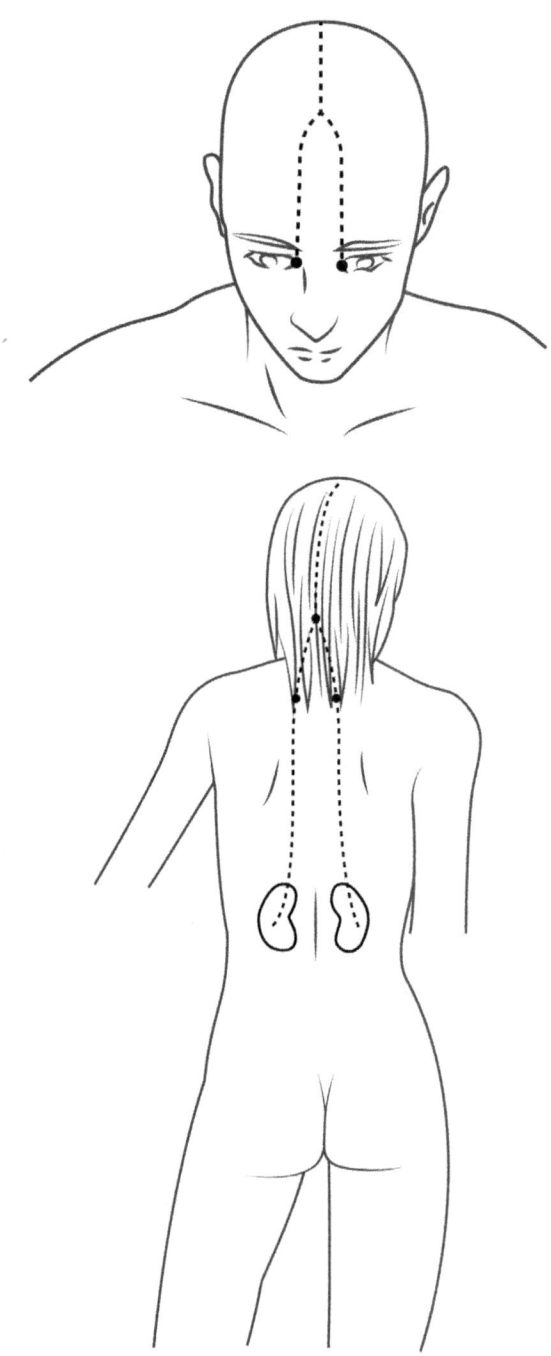

Figure 5.2: Du Mai

There is a curiosity or drive that will initiate the desire for more independence, moving more and more away from the dependency of others. Instead of being carried the child will want to "do it themselves," seeking to walk when they can. I am touched by the expression of the Du Mai every time I see a child pushing their own stroller. It makes me giggle and I have this overwhelming desire to pull out the pom-poms and cheer them on. Give me a "D," give me a "U," give me an "M-A-I!" Goooooooo Du Mai! They are moving away from their home base (yin) in order to learn from personal experience.

DU MAI AND LOSS OF INNOCENCE

The assertion of the Du Mai is a step towards individuation and is therefore accompanied by a loss of innocence. As the toddler engages the world around them they may find some aspects of the world are unsafe, cruel or difficult. Their previously idyllic world now includes experiences that alter their perceptions of it. In a healthy child, a temporary return to yin (mother) for comfort is enough to remind the child that love and support is readily available. This then revives the need for exploration once again.

In a child who lacks the strength in the Du Mai, retreat, avoidance or withdrawal may take over. When the Du Mai is weak or if there is an overly concerned or fearful mother (Ren Mai) there can be a desire in the child to avoid pain, failure and judgment. These children tend to limit their exploration of the world. They tend to have difficulty learning new things, preferring that someone else do it for them. Children who have not been fortunate enough to have the safety of the maternal matrix may approach the exploration of the world in a fearful or limited way. They may be clingy and prefer to stay close to whatever or whoever they perceive as the source of safety. These children may be slow to walk, prefer to be carried, have delayed speech or difficulty potty training and they may be fearful in the face of new things or people.

DU MAI AND EXPLORATION

This outward investigation is a necessary stage of development. Children must have the opportunity to try and fail and try again. They need to have people around them who will encourage them to attempt and explore. The expansion outward gives the baby the opportunity to try new things and develop new skills. This exploration is responsible for a child's developing sense of identity as a separate individual who can develop mastery of the world around them. If this developmental stage is supported, then children develop confidence in their ability to accomplish the tasks that their curiosity pushes them towards. This is not an abandonment of the Ren Mai but rather an essential movement towards finding a balance between the two.

Children with a healthy maternal matrix will test their limits freely knowing that they can easily return to the mother should things get uncomfortable. Children with healthy father role models are encouraged and inspired to experience new things because they can see the confidence and enthusiasm in their father's eyes.

Sometimes, children who lack maternal resources will respond in the opposite manner. Having no sense of safety or comfort to draw on, they may over-extend themselves into the world in a reckless way because they do not know the security of the Ren. They live a "hard-knocks" life, constantly having to overcome the fact that the world is a difficult place. Early on these children might be celebrated as "fearless" but the truth is that they are wounded. Without the unconditional love of the Ren Mai, they do not realize that their life is precious. They are not aware of how much their life matters. So they cannot fully know the consequences of their reckless behavior.

OVERCOMING A CONTROLLING REN MAI

Children who are too tightly bonded to the Ren due to over-controlling mothers or mothers who are themselves fearful may have great difficulty separating. If their early attempts are thwarted by a fearful or controlling mom they may give up their need for exploration. If, however, the Du Mai is strong enough constitutionally or if the father supplies the energy of the Du Mai sufficiently then maybe the child will rebel against the over-bonding and try to separate. This driving force of yang may be so strong that it even causes the child to separate too soon. Some children are gifted a curriculum from the Chong Mai that causes them to assert their need for independence through the Du Mai very early on.

DU MAI AND THE DRIVE FOR EARLY INDEPENDENCE

My son was a very active baby and an early walker. He was very active in the womb and from the time he was born, I would lay him against my chest (Ren Mai) and almost immediately he would begin to "inchworm" his way up and over my shoulder to my back (Du Mai). I would pull him back down to my chest and he would begin inching upwards once again.

He weaned himself at seven months and it became very apparent to me that he would prefer a sippy-cup to go than to nurse in the safety of his mother's arms. So, reluctantly I admit, I let him go. He didn't really crawl. He just got up and started walking. This impulse to walk early comes through the Du Mai from the Chong Mai. It is a constitutional predisposition.

Although he has always been independent and very bright, he had some homework issues in school. This turned out, in part, to be a vision problem that affected his ability to read out loud and comprehend what he was reading. Because he didn't crawl he developed a blind spot in his field of vision right down the center, between his eyes. His rush to independence did not allow his brain to develop in the center where information crosses from one side to the other (yin and yang). The eyes are one of the areas where the Du and Ren meet. This was corrected with vision therapy. Interestingly, the vision therapy involved a lot of time jumping up and down on a rebounder, which in theory should activate the fourth trajectory of the Chong and increase the ability to stimulate that area of the brain that missed out on the chance to develop because he did not crawl.

This early streak of independence definitely had something to do with the relationship between his eyes and his brain. Of course, my opinion about his early independence has a slight bias because I would have been happy to extend his time in the maternal matrix for just a little bit longer but his will is strong and he knows what he wants.

MOTIVATION FOR INDIVIDUATION

This early childhood transition between the Ren and the Du has a tremendous impact on how people individuate. It dictates how they make their way in the world. Healthy individuals need a balance of Ren and Du energy. They need someone in their lives to teach them how to bond in a healthy manner but they also need someone in their lives to help them engage and activate the motive force needed to explore the world.

As an adult you can think of the Du Mai as that which motivates you. Are you a person who likes to explore the world around you? Are you interested in new things and new ideas? The Du Mai governs the spine and upright posture. Can you stand up for yourself? Do you have a spine? How do you deal with authority? Do you need others to create structure for your life or does it make you angry when people tell you where to go and what to do?

In a healthy childhood we are given an opportunity to spread our wings and fly. Our parents may allow us to fall but usually it is in small ways so that we can learn from our failures without injuring ourselves too badly. Over time we learn what we are capable of and it is hoped we are brave enough to keep trying to learn new things.

DU MAI AND COURAGE

If the Du Mai energy is depleted or constitutionally weak then our will is compromised and we may not feel as if we can accomplish anything. We can lose our self-respect and we may be prone to apathy or cowardice. It is interesting that cowardice is often portrayed in images as the coward having a big yellow stripe down the center of the back and to be cowardly one is said to have "tucked tail and run." The strength of the spine and the uprightness of posture is mediated by the relationship between Du-4, Du-14 and Du-20. If we have a solid upright posture we are much more likely to have the courage and will to make our way in the world.

DU MAI EXCESS

If there is an excess in the Du Mai it may show itself in physiological symptoms like seizures or rigidity in the spine. That rigidity may also show up emotionally or cognitively. A person with excess in the Du Mai may be resistant to compromise. They may see things in a black-and-white kind of way. They may be more extroverted in nature or more comfortable with thinking rather than feeling. Heat is common in excess patterns of the Du Mai, which may result in anger management issues or if the heat stirs wind you might see impulsive or risky behavior with a clear disregard for the consequences of that behavior. This is action without due consideration.

The Du Mai is the vessel that holds you upright, standing tall and able to make your way in the world. It gives you the courage to face your fears and the will to move through them. It provides you with motive force.

DU MAI PATHWAY

The primary pathway of the Du Mai begins in the lower jiao in the same place as the Chong and Ren. It descends and emerges into the region of the perineum, turns towards the back of the body ascending the posterior midline to the head and turns towards the front of the body following the anterior midline of the face to meet the Ren Mai inside the mouth at Du-28. This branch enters and exits the brain, affecting neurological and cognitive function. The Du Mai has a branch that overlays the Ren Mai pathway, which once again reminds us of the inter-connectedness of yin and yang. This branch gives the Du Mai a connection to the heart. The third and fourth trajectories connect the prenatal source of yang to the postnatal expression of yang through the Urinary Bladder channel and the kidneys. The intersection points for these connections are UB-23, UB-12 and UB-1.

A weakness in the yang of the Du Mai may lead to an inability to maintain an upright posture and have the courage and will to engage life. An excess in the Du Mai may lead to an inability to contain yang, causing anger management issues or impulsive behavior.

Common conditions treated by the Du Mai

- Neurological conditions, especially those that affect consciousness and cognition like fainting, seizures and memory loss.

- Hypofunction associated with Kidney or Heart yang deficiency.

- Gynecological problems associated with Kidney yang deficiency like infertility and hypothalamic amenorrhea.

- Wind conditions: both interior and exterior wind (wind-stroke and wind-cold).

- Spinal problems, especially stiffness, with an inability to bend forwards and backwards.

- Dysfunction in the lower burner especially when associated with qi sinking or failure of yang to consolidate (hemorrhoids and incontinence).

- Aching in the head, neck or back.

THE PERFECT PARENT

As we leave the first ancestry and begin to take a look at how we use the resources this ancestry gives us, I would like to say something about parenting. I have just spent three chapters discussing what happens to us if our parents do not give us everything we need. I have spoken about how our ability to pursue meaning in life is directly correlated with the failures of our caregivers. So now I would like to defend parents. Although you will undoubtedly have a patient or two who suffered horrible abuse at the hands of their parents or grandparents, most of us had parents who wanted to do what was best for us. There is no excuse for violence or child abuse, but most of our parents wanted to help us turn into functioning members of society. They loved us to the best of their ability. Here is the truth about parenting: there is no rule book or tool kit. When you take on the job of parenting you are basically winging it and hoping, sometimes praying, for the best. The job of parenting is to make yourself redundant. If you have done an adequate job your children will grow up and leave you to live their own lives. That's a little like ripping your heart out of your chest, giving it legs and then watching it walk away. It's a tough job and the only training you ever get is the example your parents set for you.

It is important to remember that your parents were once children and if they didn't get everything they needed then it is unlikely that they will have the capacity to give those things to you. As parents we swear when we have children that we will do better than our parents. We assure ourselves that we can parent differently than they did and then one day something comes out of our mouths and we groan. We know that what we just said is almost verbatim something that our parents said to us. We have become our parents.

Fortunately, we are not just our parents and if we choose we can learn to parent more consciously. We can stop blaming our parents for our weaknesses and failures. We can accept the reality of our childhoods and then remember that we are now adults and one of the best things about being an adult is that we have a choice. One of the greatest gifts you can give to your parents and yourself is to forgive them and thank them for doing the best they could do.

CHAPTER 6

THE WEI VESSELS

aka: Yin and Yang Linking Vessels

As the first ancestry of the 8 EV, the Chong, Du and Ren contain all of the resources we have been gifted for our journey in life. We are then responsible for the choices we make that support or direct those resources. We can use them for growth, development and health, or not. We are capable of learning from our experiences and when those experiences are challenging or difficult we can adapt how we do things based on what we have learned over time.

The Yin and Yang Wei Mai are the vessels that influence how we use the resources given to us through the first ancestry. The Wei vessels are able to do this in part because of their ability to "link" the yin channels together and the yang channels together. This linking creates an avenue for communication and a system through which the resources of the Ren and Du can be distributed. Over time, we have an opportunity to learn how best to use our resources, expending, conserving and replenishing when appropriate.

This capacity for distribution of resources becomes more noticeable when we are faced with challenges or transitions in life. The 8 EV govern the cycles of growth and development. Those cycles transition every seven years in females and every eight years in males. As we move from one cycle to the next we must adapt how we use our resources. For example, menstruating women have a different relationship to their blood than post-menopausal women. In menstruating women the goal is to build enough resources to be able to support a pregnancy or if there is no pregnancy to then release that blood without suffering a deficit. In post-menopausal women the focus is on preservation of yin (blood) and maintaining a healthy balance between yin and yang. So, the menses stop and the ebb and flow of blood now transitions into a consistent effort to conserve the yin. We can see the impact on the emotions during the transitions. In menstruating women emotions ebb and flow with the blood. Women can often clock their cycles based on their emotions. In the peri-menopausal transition there is more chaos as the body tries to move from the cyclic changes of menstruation to the conservation mode of menopause. This is a bit like rewiring a house, moving from alternating current to direct current. The alternating current may be a little unpredictable but emotion during this stage is more temporary and dissipates as blood leaves the body. In the direct current of menopause, for the first time since childhood women experience very directed emotion that doesn't ebb and flow but rather must be processed consciously. As we work to conserve yin (blood) the emotions we experience are often the driving force in how we pursue our purpose in the latter years of our lives. In between these two currents we have the chaos of transition. We need a system that helps us to make use of those resources in a new way, a system that helps us to adapt to the transition. The Wei vessels are that system.

In some ways we may think of the Wei vessels as the vessels of aging. The resources needed in puberty for instance are different than the ones needed in middle age. In puberty the resources are directed towards individuation and exploration. There is an outward directed energy that is meant to help us gather the information and experience we need to become who we are meant to be as adults. By middle age what we often see is energy directed towards letting go. If we have children, they are getting ready to leave and live their own lives. This means that life can be simpler and we need less stuff. The resources of middle age are also often directed more towards self-care. We are learning that we can no longer get away with extravagant use of resources. We cannot eat or drink the way we used to when we were younger. We have to conserve more and perhaps be more discerning in how we direct our resources. How people handle the aging process and the allocation of resources is directly related to the proper functioning of the Wei vessels.

During times of stress or change we also adjust the usage of our resources. When we move to a new home, change jobs, get married, get divorced, have children or have to deal with a life crisis like illness, we may require more support from our resources. Which resources we use may be a determining factor in how successfully we negotiate the challenges. The proper functioning of the Wei vessels helps us to "hold it together" in the face of change. So, when we are resistant to change there is often an imbalance in the Wei Mai.

In their capacity to distribute these resources over time the Wei vessels become a record of our history. They are in some ways the representation of our story, our biography. The Yin Wei records the events that have occurred in our lives and how those events have changed the substance or structure of who we are. The Yang Wei records the actions we have taken to create the life we currently have. My esteemed teacher, Jeffrey Yuen often uses the analogy of woven cloth as a metaphor for the Wei vessels. The cloth itself and the patterns or images on the cloth represent the Yin Wei and the actions taken by the weaver to weave the cloth represents the Yang Wei. When we look back on our lives we can see how the actions we have taken have resulted in the person we are today. We can also see how events in our lives have shaped us, changed us.

Our history often affects our perception of the future. If we have imbalance in the Wei vessels we spend too much time and effort on what has happened before and what may happen in the future. We are not able to be present in the moment. If we are stuck in the past, *longing* for what has been, the Yin Wei may be imbalanced. If we are fearful of moving forward, *immobilized* by a fear of the unknown, the Yang Wei may be imbalanced.

Fantasy or magical thinking, resistance to change or obsession with what has not yet happened keeps us out of the present moment and that mindset requires resources to thrive. Qi and blood are consumed by living in the past or fearing the future and eventually those resources decline. Since the body is built for self-preservation, it responds to the loss of resources by creating stagnation to try to stop the loss. This stagnation is then responsible for pain and suffering.

THE YIN WEI MAI

The Yin Wei has a strong association with ying qi (nutritive qi) and blood. By linking yin, it governs the interior terrain of the body. It connects the resources of the Ren Mai to the postnatal yin channels. Through this connection we can use the prenatal yin of the Ren Mai when we need it but we can also support the prenatal yin by healthy generation of postnatal yin. This link allows us to return yin to its origin.

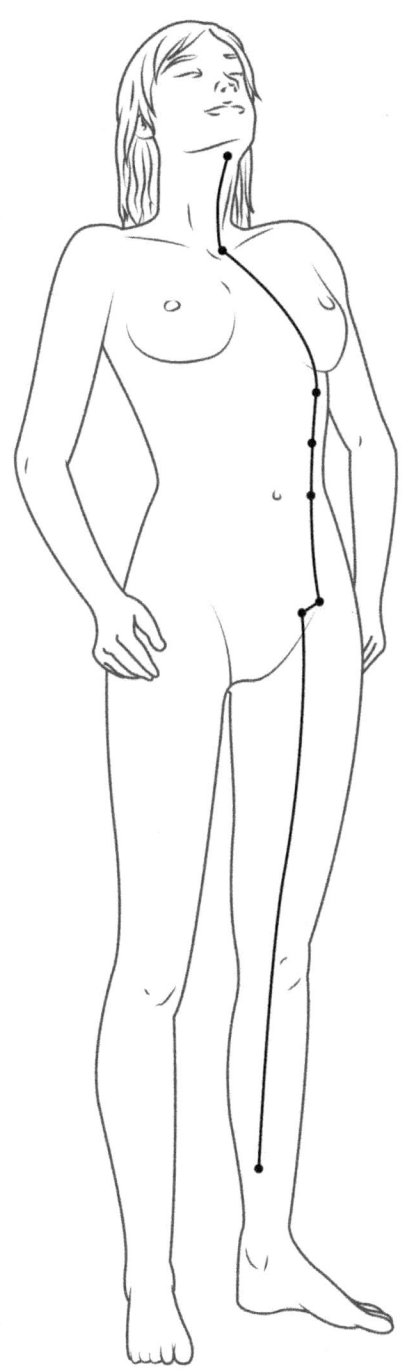

Figure 6.1: Yin Wei

YIN WEI AND HEART PAIN

As we move through the cycles of aging we must go from the safety and love of the maternal matrix (Ren Mai) out into the world. Experiences in the world are not always happy or satisfying. In fact, some of the most powerful experiences we have in life are the ones that are disappointing or frustrating. When the Yin Wei is functioning well we are able to take those disappointments and learn from them in a way that we are content with what we have learned. We understand that those experiences have helped us to become a better version of ourselves. When there is pathology in the Yin Wei, those disappointments take us out of the present moment and we begin to obsess about those events and we feel discontented. We become unhappy about the state of our being-ness. Resources, especially blood, are consumed by this dissatisfaction and that results in stagnation, which then produces the most common symptom of Yin Wei pathology: heart pain. People with Yin Wei pathology have emotional pain that creates suffering in all aspects of living. For how can one feel successful in life, in love, in work if one is not content with who they are?

YIN WEI AND SUPPRESSION

The Yin Wei is the vessel that is most responsible for the mediation of our emotional bodies. When there is pathology, patients experience anxiety, shame, guilt, unfulfilled yearning. They feel broken-hearted. They suffer from an emotional state that makes them feel out of control in their lives. They may feel unable to achieve the future they want because they are still stuck in the memories of a traumatic or unhappy past. This unhappiness or obsession with the past consumes the blood and deprives the shen (mind/spirit) of adequate nourishment. Which, of course, leads to further emotional distress.

These patients often feel that everything would be better if they could rewrite their history. They are consumed by the "what ifs." "What if I had been born at a different time?" "What if I had different parents?" "What if I didn't have to move after my parents got divorced?" They suffer from anxiety based on the reality of their past and their inability to overcome it.

In some cases patients are unable to remember their past because they have repressed the memories. They may know they are suffering but they may not actually understand why. Whatever trauma or traumas they experienced earlier in their lives were so overwhelming that they were unable to deal with them or overcome the feelings around it. So, in order to survive they had to repress those memories.

Many repressed memories are pushed down into the Dai Mai, which we will discuss in later chapters. In the case of the Yin Wei often what we see are repressed or partially suppressed memories. The Pericardium supports the suppression as a means for self-preservation. Although the memories have been forgotten, the feelings associated with the trauma continue causing anxiety, discontent or fear, but the patient has no frame of reference for the feelings. This repression or suppression may occur in a way that we consciously choose to forget the upsetting event or we may unconsciously choose to forget. Sometimes we only forget certain aspects of the memories or the feelings associated with the memories. In some cases people often have reframed the events in their minds to be less traumatic by a process of selective memory. It is common for people to focus on the good times in their past hoping to drown out the bad memories. But sometimes we can actually create false memories to overcome the bad. A person's internal reality is no longer in alignment with the reality of the past.

YIN WEI AND COMMUNICATION

As the pathway of the Yin Wei moves into the throat at Ren-22 and Ren-23 we can see difficulty in expression. Patients may have difficulty telling their story. If there is past trauma they may not be able to speak of it. This can produce a tension or tightness in the throat. This may be severe enough to be diagnosed as plum-pit or it could be just a sensation of holding back in the throat. This is also a type of repression where the patient may be unwilling or not ready to talk about their story. They may be unable to find the words or they may be afraid that if they tell their story the emotions may overwhelm them.

YIN WEI AND AGING

Pathology in the Yin Wei frequently results in a resistance to aging. The discontent of Yin Wei imbalance is expressed in an acute discomfort with the visible changes that occur in aging. There is anxiety related to the eventual effects of gravity and time on the body. The emotions about the sagging, wrinkling, graying of hair and, of course, my favorite, the redistribution of weight (Yin) are all intensified in Yin Wei pathology. Most of us want to age well but we don't necessarily like to be reminded of changes that occur as we age. We may struggle a little with the changes and we may increase our effort to stay youthful by modifying our lifestyle, eating better or trying a new age-defying cream or two. People with Yin Wei pathology may become obsessed with aging or anxious and desperate about what is happening to them. These people may use extreme measures to avoid the visible signs of aging. They may remember a time when they were considered valuable or admired based on their looks and they will do whatever it takes to avoid the ravages of time and go back to that youthful image. The problem with that process is there is no way to go back. So whatever temporary improvement one gets from cosmetics or surgery cannot stop time from moving on and the reality of this produces a constant state of anxiety.

YIN WEI AND DISCONTENT

In an effort to maintain communication in the interior the Yin Wei has an impact on how we feel about what is happening in our lives. When the Yin Wei functions well and is sufficiently nourished we can use our resources wisely and we are able to manage the challenges and transitions in life with ease and grace. We feel content with who we are and where we are going in life. Even when the transitions are challenging, we are able to move through the discomfort and not get stuck in the "what ifs." When we lack that self-contentment we are unable to manage life's challenges well. We become discontented with life or discontented with who we have become. We feel anxious, depressed and frustrated and our mental-emotional process may be obsessive.

Once again, this emotional distress consumes the blood and produces stagnation that results in heart pain. It also often results in other types of pain. When the spirit cannot resolve the heart pain it produces a spiritual or psychic tension that is detrimental to organ function. In an act of self-preservation this tension may be somaticized. The Yin Wei has a relationship with the Yang Wei and the distress that is accumulating in the chest and abdomen is pushed out to the exterior causing more superficial pain that is less immediately detrimental to the function of the organs. You may see this in conditions like fibromyalgia or chronic joint pain.

YIN WEI PATHWAY

The pathway of the Yin Wei begins on the medial aspect of the lower leg at Ki-9 then proceeds up the medial aspect of the leg to the abdomen intersecting Sp-13, Sp-15 and Sp-16. From here it proceeds into the chest at Lv-14 where it returns to the origin of source yin at Ren-22 and Ren-23. The pathway demonstrates the linking process by moving through three leg yin (Kidney, Spleen and Liver) and then connecting with constitutional yin

(Ren Mai), providing the connections that govern the interior terrain of emotions.

Common conditions treated by the Yin Wei

- Pain in the chest and heart region.

- Fullness or constriction in the hypochondriac region. Diaphragm constriction.

- Conditions related to blood and yin deficiency.

- Bi syndrome related to blood deficiency (numbness and tingling in the joints).

- Mental-emotional problems like depression, anxiety and restless organ syndrome (Zang Zao), especially those related to blood deficiency.

- Backache associated with emotional constraint, particularly fear, fright and sadness.

- Digestive problems: vomiting, indigestion, food sensitivities, gas and bloating.

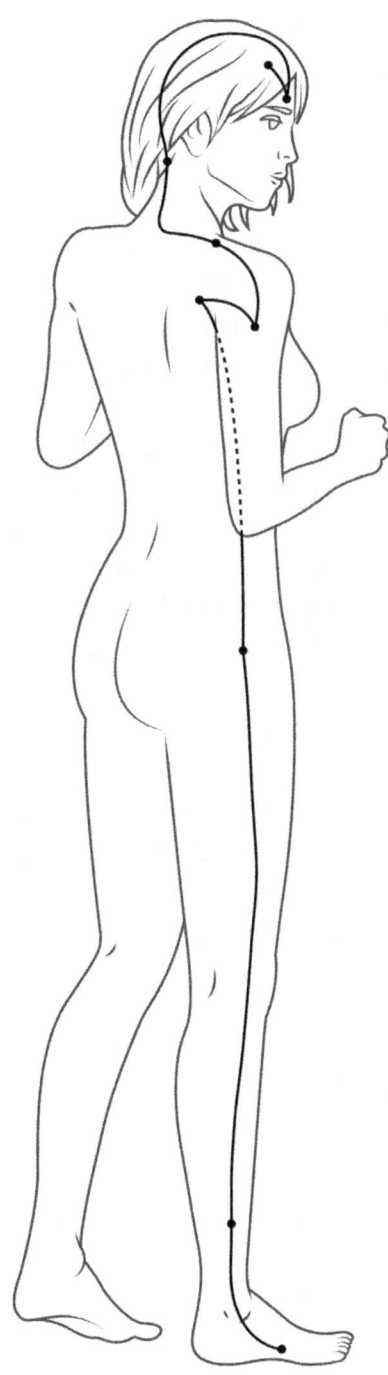

Figure 6.2: Yang Wei

THE YANG WEI MAI

The Yang Wei links all of the yang channels to the Du Mai and uses the resources of the Du Mai to take action in life. The Yang Wei links the yang channels and governs the exterior of the body. The Du Mai gives us the motive force to separate from the maternal matrix and individuate. The Yang Wei helps us decide how to use the motive force to support that individuation. The Du Mai gives us the desire to explore the world around us and the Yang Wei helps us decide what actions we will take to accomplish that exploration.

When the Yang Wei is healthy we are able to act in a socially accepted and effective manner that is beneficial to our growth and sense of well-being. Our behavior is appropriate to the circumstance and an authentic expression of who we are. If we are really angry we may feel like "acting out," using physical violence or inappropriate language to express those feelings. A healthy Yang Wei reminds us that violence might provide emotional release but ultimately it will not end with us getting what we want. We learn over time that expressing our anger by beating someone up is not socially acceptable and may result in irreparable damage to interpersonal relationships or, in some cases, jail time. With a healthy Yang Wei we can still feel and express the anger but we will do it in a way that is not detrimental to our growth or sense of self.

YANG WEI AND CONFLICT

When we have pathology in the Yang Wei we may have a fear of moving forward based on our history or experience. For instance, if we have had a serious relationship that ended badly we may be reluctant to engage in a new relationship for fear that the next relationship will inevitably end as badly as the last. Or, if we are in a committed relationship and we have an argument that escalates and causes all kinds of pain, we may stop arguing. We may do anything to avoid conflict. When this happens the anger we experience has to be displaced in order to avoid the conflict. We may swallow it down and it may express itself in physical ailments like headaches or joint pain. We may find a way to dampen down the emotion so it is less intense by drinking, eating too much or watching too much TV.

The anger may also be expressed covertly or unconsciously in the form of passive-aggressive behavior. I had a relationship many years ago with a man who had difficulty with anger. He was a very nice man who was very even-tempered. When he got angry at me he used to do laundry and shrink my sweaters. He would say he was only trying to help. He was genuinely apologetic afterwards. What he could not do was tell me he was angry. His fear of conflict made it almost impossible for him to see the possibility of healthy conflict resolution. At that time in my life, I was a big fan of conflict, which I am certain made his life much more difficult, thus I had drawers full of shrunken clothing.

This fear of moving forward is a form of resistance to change. The resistance causes stagnation, which causes heat that makes us uncomfortable. We can use this discomfort as the impetus to change or we can create dampness to muffle the discomfort. The dampness does keep the heat in check at first but then eventually it causes even more stagnation, which increases suffering. This is a Yang Wei pathology.

YANG WEI AND AGING

One of the ways that this resistance to change while aging occurs is in people who continue to act as though they are 25 even though they are long past that age. The cliché of the midlife crisis is an easy to understand example of this. This typically occurs when someone is approaching a big birthday (an important passage) like 39 or 40. The person may feel some dread about this approaching marker in time. Perhaps the person is feeling as if they are managing the emotions of this change until someone makes a seemingly innocent comment that triggers a heightened awareness of aging or shift in self-perception. "How does it feel to be one year away from the Big 4-0?" "Wow, 40, guess you are on the downhill slide now." "When are you going to start a family?" "What are you doing to prepare for your retirement?" These reminders may cause significant discord and a resistance to the inevitable. So the person unconsciously tries to recreate the feelings of youth in the hopes that the clock can be turned back. Maybe they buy a little red sports car or maybe they go out drinking when they have to be at work the next morning. They may even get divorced and start dating someone much younger as a way of trying to recapture their youth. This may temporarily distract someone from aging but eventually it fails because we cannot go backwards in time.

As is true with the Yin Wei, the Yang Wei is supposed to help us make the transitions through the seven/eight year cycles of jing. It is supposed to help us adapt during the aging process. It is supposed to help us refine our behavior as we age. This includes our behavior when we are stressed or challenged. We are supposed to learn from our previous experiences. Most of us know by the time that we are adults that temper tantrums are not an effective way to build relationships. We have learned this from the consequences of our actions.

Carl Jung speaks of the archetype of the Puer/Puella, the Eternal Child. Think Peter Pan. This resistance to aging is based on the memory of a time when we were younger and happier. A time perhaps when we felt as if we had more influence or more potential. A time when we had big dreams that were not yet dashed by failure. This archetype is what pathology in the Yang Wei looks like. We focus on that happier time in the past, refusing or unable to see the options available to us in the future. Believing that nothing that is coming in the days and years ahead can be as good as the happy memories of the past.

YANG WEI AND SHAO YANG

The Yang Wei has a very strong relationship to the Gall Bladder and shao yang. Decisions need to be made about how we will use the resources of the Du Mai. What actions will keep us moving through time? This relationship can also be evident in Yang Wei pathology through judgment and blame. People who have Yang Wei pathology frequently are disappointed with their lot in life. They may feel as though they have somehow settled for the life they have. It is not uncommon for them to blame others for their circumstances. This Gall Bladder connection often shows up as depression or lacking momentum or a sense of direction in life. They may feel as though they have never found their passion in life or have never mastered anything. They often cannot focus on one thing long enough to master it. They seem to have trouble prioritizing and are distracted easily. They have a history of having their fingers in too many pies, hoping to find the right pie but never quite finding it. This is very disappointing and makes relationships or socialization difficult. It is not unlike the movement of a chicken with its head removed from its body. There is significant movement but it is chaotic and lacking in purpose. It is movement that is going nowhere.

YANG WEI AND SELF-SABOTAGE

People with Yang Wei pathology are prone to self-defeating or self-sabotaging behavior. Even when they know a behavior didn't work in the past they will continue the behavior and somehow hope for a different result. They may have suffered a terrible loss and then they withdrew. Even though that withdrawal may not have been constructive, every time they feel a loss they will continue to withdraw. Another example of this would be a person who lashes out physically when they are angry or afraid. Even though that has never been a successful behavior it will be their automatic response when those same feelings recur.

It is common for some with Yang Wei pathology to be immobilized by fear. They may be stuck in the "freeze" mode of the sympathetic nervous system response. When they are afraid they do nothing. Once again this is a fear of the future. Ultimately this is a fear of death. It is the inability to negotiate the ultimate transition. Treating the Yang Wei can be very helpful in patients who are having difficulty accepting their impending passage from end-stage diseases. When you can create balance in the Wei vessels both Yin and Yang people may find they can face the ultimate transition with more ease, less fear and the peace of mind that comes with acceptance.

These are people who lack the capacity for right action at least in part because their yang qi is scattered by fear or impeded by dampness. This often leaves them feeling as though nothing can ever go right. It leaves them feeling as though real success is impossible to achieve—that doing nothing is better than being disappointed one more time.

YANG WEI PATHWAY

The pathway of the Yang Wei begins at UB-63, which is the xi-cleft point of the Urinary Bladder channel. As it circles around the lateral malleolus it rises up the lateral aspect of the leg to intersect with GB-35, which is the xi-cleft point of the Yang Wei. It is interesting to note that the first two points on the Yang Wei are xi-cleft points, as this vessel's most common emotional pathology is a "stuckness" that is caused by our need to dampen down so that we cannot move through transition. The pathway rises up the lateral aspect of the leg (shao yang) to connect at GB-29 in the hip region. From here it rises up the flank to the shoulder connecting with LI-14, SI-10 and SJ-14, crossing GB-21 to ascend to the nape of the neck at GB-20 where it follows the GB channel to GB-13 and GB-14 where it turns and goes back to the nape through GB-15 to GB-19 where it returns to its origins of source yang at Du-16 and Du-15.

For those of you who have done some other reading on the 8 EV you may notice that this pathway is not the same as some of the others you have seen. There are a number of alternate pathways. What is most significant in the Yang Wei pathway on the head is the preponderance of Gall Bladder points and the return to the Du Mai at Du-15 and Du-16. In the pathway of the Yang Qiao that is coming up there is more influence on the head from the Urinary Bladder and Stomach points. I see this as the Yang Wei representing the flexibility and adaptability (shao yang) necessary to face change in the most effect manner. The Yang Wei is about seeing your options and having the courage to overcome your fears in order to face the next challenge in your life.

Common conditions treated by the Yang Wei

- Conditions that affect the circulation of Wei qi (defensive qi). Exterior wind, shao yang disorders, shivering and Bi syndrome.

- Ear problems especially those related to exterior attacks, shao yang disorders, Liver and Gall Bladder patterns.

- Headaches along the Gall Bladder channel.

- Back, shoulder and hip pain (pain along the lateral aspect of the body).

- Dyspnea with raised shoulders.

CHAPTER 7

THE QIAO VESSELS

aka: Yin and Yang Heel Vessels, Yin and Yang
Walker Vessels, Yin and Yang Elevators

The Yin and Yang Qiao vessels both originate in the region of the ankles and they intersect at UB-1 at the inner canthus of the eyes. These pathways are why the Qiao vessels can be thought of as vessels of perspective and stance. In the process of individuation we move away from the safety of our parents and families and we begin to take a stand in the world as individuals. When we do that we develop our own vision of the world around us. The lens through which we see the world is based on how we see ourselves. We learn to examine our sense of self as we move away from the bond or control of the maternal matrix (Ren Mai) to begin to establish our own sense of self and our own sense of values. We begin to see the world around us based on that vision. We have the opportunity to look at the world and ourselves through the eyes of an individuated adult.

These two vessels balance the relationship between insight and exploration. The Wei vessels (Yin and Yang Wei) are about how we use the resources from the first ancestry (Chong, Ren and Du) as we age, over time. Whereas, the Qiao vessels govern how we use those resources right here, right now, in the present moment. They govern our capacity to use our resources appropriately from day to day. The Wei vessels are how we deal with changes or transitions that occur over time and the Qiao vessels are about how we occupy our bodies and the space around us in the present. With their connection to the eyes they also help us manage the daily cycles of yin and yang (night and day) by opening and closing the eyes.

YIN QIAO MAI

The Yin Qiao creates an opportunity for self-illumination. It allows us to turn our vision inward and expand our self-knowledge, self-awareness and consciousness. In short, it gives us the capacity for deeper insight. This is about the ability to see ourselves with clarity in the present moment and be comfortable with what we see. The foot aspect of this vessel's path (Ki-2, Ki-6 and Ki-8) also allows us to take a stand, in this moment, in the society we choose to engage. How easy is it for you to take a stand at your job or in your family? Can you take a stand with your friends when you don't agree? Do you trust yourself enough to hold your own when people challenge you and your beliefs?

The Yin Qiao, like the Yin Wei is an offspring of Primal Yin (Ren Mai). If we have not been taught self-love or an appreciation for self then how do we "see" ourselves? If our own Ren Mai has been damaged by lack of care or obstructed by the care of an obsessive mother then how does that affect the "stand" we take in society? Are we able to be at ease with who we are or do we need to deny or suppress who we are to feel accepted by others? Can we trust that we are deserving of love and acceptance?

If the Ren Mai has not supplied us with a sense of self-love then the Yin Qiao will begin to stagnate. This stagnation may present itself with a sense of us not being comfortable with who we are. If the stagnation is severe enough we will be overwhelmed with self-loathing. Even if it is not severe, our place in society may be marked by an unconscious need to demonstrate in any number of ways that we are worthy because we do not trust that we are indeed worthy. We will look for outside validation of our value.

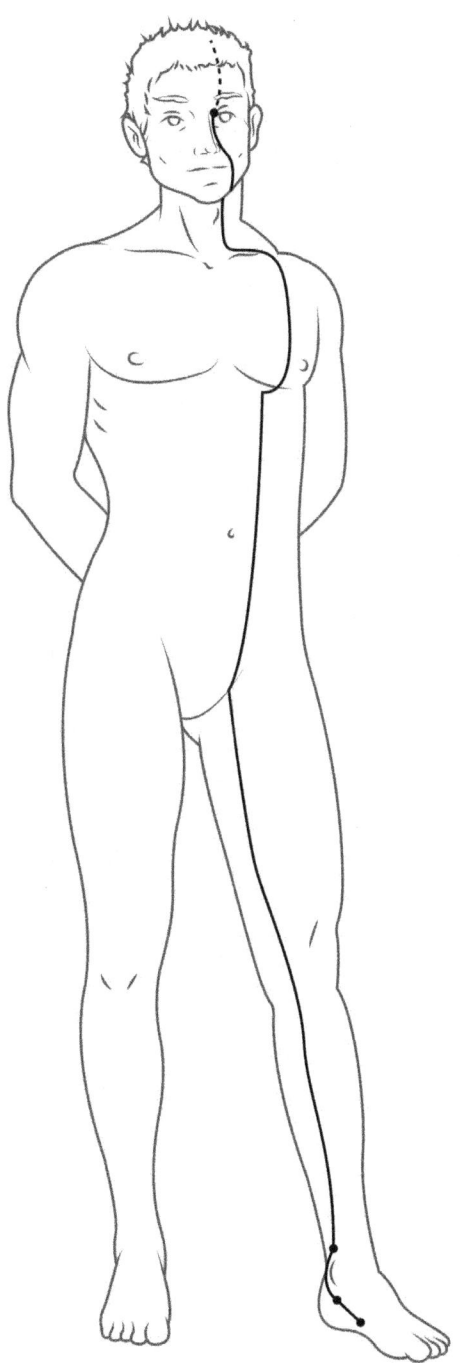

Figure 7.1: Yin Qiao

STASIS OF YIN

Physiologically, the Yin Qiao is used to treat accumulations in the abdomen. It treats stagnation and stasis of yin (blood, phlegm and dampness). In Yin Qiao pathology there may be palpable masses in the abdomen or there may be accumulation obstructing function in the abdomen. Imagine if you were told over and over again in both words and deeds that you were "*less than*." Imagine, beginning in childhood, you were made to feel wrong for simply existing. In order to survive the feelings that come from the words and actions of those we love, trust or admire we may try to push those feelings away from our heart, away from our consciousness. To keep those feelings from returning to consciousness, we wrap them up in yin (blood and body fluids). That way when we look inward those feelings are veiled by the yin and therefore they are less immediately hurtful. The veil of yin blurs and softens the intensity of the hurt so that we are able to continue living.

Of course, there is a cost for that distancing. The stagnation or masses created by this self-preservation mechanism can be physically painful and they can disrupt organ function. It is also costly in terms of our resources. It takes a lot of qi and yin to maintain the veil. Patients with Yin Qiao stagnation develop conditions like fibroids, hernias, abdominal and low back pain and genital pain, and they are also vulnerable to parasitic infestation (Gu). From a CM perspective we know that parasites prefer cold-damp (yin) environments. From a psycho-emotional point of view, the feelings of "less than" create a vacuum, a "for rent" sign that allows the parasites to take hold.

YIN QIAO AND INTERNAL ALIGNMENT

The Yin Qiao pathway begins in the medial arch of the foot, in the region of Ki-6 and Ki-2. A healthy foot arch leads to good structural alignment, which then maintains the integrity of the musculoskeletal system. If the foot arch is balanced and stable then everything else from the knees through the hips, spine and head will all align in a way that supports stability, balance and ease of movement. It might then be said that a healthy stance in life leads to internal alignment, which maintains the integrity of the self in the present moment. When we are grounded in an acceptance of self we can more easily take our place in society knowing that our lives have meaning. We can trust that we will attract people into our lives who will accept us and we will not be weighed down or wounded by those who cannot see us clearly. This acceptance of self in the present moment allows us to negotiate the world around us from a place of trust and clear insight.

When we are internally aligned we are much better able to take right action in the here and now. When the Yin Qiao is in a state of excess (stagnation) the Yang Qiao is deficient. This can be easily seen in the most notable musculoskeletal symptoms of the Qiao vessels. When there is tension or spasm in the medial aspect of the leg (excess Yin Qiao) there will be flaccidity in the lateral aspect. When there is tension in the lateral aspect (excess Yang Qiao) there will be flaccidity in the medial aspect of the leg. Since the Yang Qiao governs locomotion, the tension or stagnation in the Yin Qiao makes it quite difficult to take action in the moment. If one is able to take action in this state, the action is often not in alignment with who we are.

YIN QIAO AND WITHDRAWAL

When there is stagnation in the Yin Qiao we feel oppressed by the accumulation. We are weighed down by the hurts of the past and the accompanying sense of unworthiness. We may want to withdraw from the world around us. The healthy desire for the Yang Qiao to extend outwards and explore the world is impeded by the stagnation of yin. Stagnation of yin affects the eyes, making them heavy and difficult to open. Patients withdraw by sleeping more and are not refreshed by that sleep. They may sleep their lives away because when they are sleeping they are not hurting.

NARCISSISM AND THE YIN QIAO

This movement inward and away from engaging the world may also present in some cases as narcissism. Patients may become overly focused on the self, limiting their ability to see their place in the world around them. In a way, they may move into a place of thinking they are the center of the universe, becoming more separated from their need to engage others. They may become obsessed with their own needs and desires, disregarding the needs of others. It becomes "all about me." They become so veiled by the yin they cannot see how destructive they have become in their desire to make themselves feel better about who they are.

YIN QIAO AND ILLUMINATION

The potential of the Yin Qiao is the capacity to shed light on the darkest corner of the Self so that we may learn to more fully accept who we are. When the darkness predominates, we live unconsciously and become unwilling victims of those parts of ourselves we have not yet been able to embrace fully. If we do not know that we have a tendency to be selfish then we will be shocked, hurt or disappointed that others accuse us of being so. If we do not know that we hold within us a deep sense of emptiness or loneliness then when others suggest that we are overly needy we will not understand. We will not realize that our actions are being driven by that loneliness.

We cannot change what we cannot see. Once we can see who we are then we have a choice. As each aspect of who we are is illuminated we can then decide if we will live our lives from that aspect or if we will choose to live our lives from a more wholly integrated place. If we can see the darker aspects of who we are through the illumination provided by the Yin Qiao then we have a choice. Once we see those aspects of our Self then we can choose if those darker aspects are useful in the pursuit of our purpose. If we decide after the insight that they are not then we can consciously begin to develop virtues or behaviors that will support our growth. The more we learn about ourselves the more choice we have.

YIN QIAO AND SWALLOWING THE TRUTH

The Yin Qiao pathway passes through the throat (St-12 and St-9) on its way to the eyes (UB-1). Sometimes when we look into the deep recesses of our being we can have difficulty swallowing the truth of what we see. Physiologically this may manifest as difficulty swallowing, tightness or pain in the throat, goiter and chronic lymph swelling in the region of the neck and clavicle. Once again this is an example of how the body uses yin to muffle the pain. Treating the Yin Qiao for this type of yin accumulation in the throat is a way of supporting the patient while they struggle with self-acceptance. This type of tension is often seen in adults who were told early in life that "children should be seen and not heard" or perhaps they have been told over and over again that they don't know what they are talking about. At some point (usually unconsciously) they hold back on speaking up for fear of being reminded that what they have to say has no value. This then creates the tension in the throat region. They may have great difficulty speaking their truth or standing up for themselves.

SUICIDE AND THE YIN QIAO

Sometimes the pain and suffering is more than the Yin Qiao can absorb or veil. We may develop suicidal tendencies as a way of dealing with this pain. When we look inside we see nothing but darkness, suffering and a sense of hopelessness and this may make death seem like an avenue for relief. Nowadays we often hear of young people who attempt suicide after years of bullying. Beaten down day after day by the words and actions of others they begin to see suicide as a viable form of self-defense. They may see it as the only option left for ending the torment. The abuse is so great they cannot generate enough yin to muffle the pain so they make a decision to end it all and then they begin to work towards gathering enough yang to complete the task. Treating the Yin Qiao in patients with suicidal tendencies can help them to trust that they can survive this moment—that things are not hopeless. It can help them to see that they are not worthless and that they have people in their lives who love them. Just to be clear, I am not suggesting that you should treat patients who are suicidal without first referring out for the appropriate mental health care. What I am suggesting is that if you can free up the stagnation in suicidal patients by using the Yin Qiao, this might aid whatever therapeutic process they are receiving. You may be able to give those patients an internal sense that they have what it takes to continue, to survive and even to defeat their tormentors by having a meaningful life.

BUFFERING AND WEIGHT GAIN

A word about obesity and the Yin Qiao. Obesity is a very complex health concern. Patients who are obese are not patients who are simply eating too much. Most obese patients have many factors that have led them to their current health. There may be a genetic influence, hormonal imbalances, lifestyle issues and a deep-seated emotional component. For patients to improve their health they must adequately address all of these issues. This can be very challenging because body fat is stagnating yin and stagnating yin serves a purpose. It provides a buffer against the judgment of others and a deep sense of unworthiness. Society in general is not kind to obese people. It has little compassion for the suffering of those who are obese. It does little to accommodate those who are more greatly buffered than the average person.

It may seem counterintuitive to those who have never been really overweight but when you are overweight, even though you are larger in size, you actually become less visible. What most people see when they look at you is not you, but the protection of yin. They see the buffer but they do not know it is a buffer. Although it is painful to be judged by others for your physical appearance, this decrease in visibility actually feels safer and less exposed. To lose the weight is to lose the protection. The weight loss increases the visibility and therefore the vulnerability. Patients who are overweight must negotiate the feelings associated with that vulnerability. They must learn to be comfortable enough with who they are so that when others see and judge them they can still hold on to their own image of self. If they cannot achieve a level of self-acceptance then if they do lose weight it will frequently come back with a few extra pounds to account for the latest discomfort.

There is no doubt that when a person is overweight they know they are overweight. They do not need someone else to tell them they need to lose weight. Yin Qiao treatments can help these patients to see themselves more clearly and accept who they are. These treatments can help them to trust that they are so much more than their current physical status. They can learn to recognize that they are worthy of love, worthy of kindness and worthy of self-care, and that this would be true regardless of their weight. These treatments can also help them to trust themselves enough that their ability to feel safer in the world increases. The need for the buffer lessens.

The illumination of the Yin Qiao helps to create an internal vision of self that is stronger, more resilient and more in alignment with our spirit and our purpose. This vision then overcomes the judgment of others and as a result, the need for buffering.

YIN QIAO PATHWAY

The pathway points from the foot at Ki-2, Ki-6 and Ki-8 to the throat at St-12 and St-9, rising up the eyes at UB-1. From here it enters the brain and in some texts the pathway is said to emerge at GB-20, connecting it for a second time to the Yang Qiao. The lower portion of the pathway shows us the importance of the arch of the foot in developing internal alignment and a healthy stance. The upper portion demonstrates the significance of insight in developing a sense of self.

Common conditions treated by the Yin Qiao

- Eye diseases.

- Somnolence (desire to close the eyes).

- Abdominal pain with masses.

- Wei syndrome with flaccidity in the lateral aspect of the leg with tightness in the medial aspect of the leg.

- Urinary problems associated with excess (dampness, qi stagnation and blood stasis).

- Obstetric problems: prolonged labor, placental retention and unilateral abdominal pain post-partum. Problems associated with excess, especially blood stasis.

- Obstruction in the lower burner: Shan conditions, leukorrhea, genital pain and hypogastric pain.

- Night-time epilepsy.

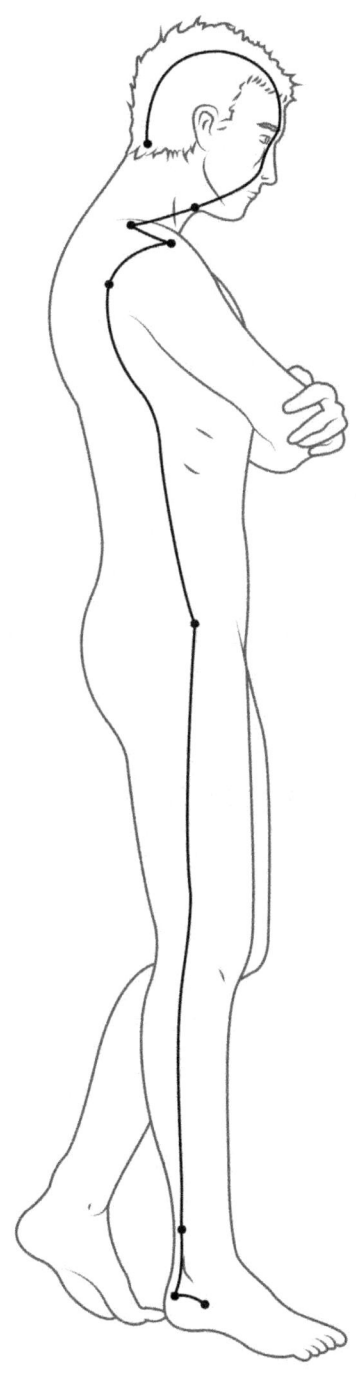

Figure 7.2: Yang Qiao

YANG QIAO

The Yang Qiao is about locomotion. This vessel is what determines how we engage the world around us in the present moment. Can we clearly see the world around us and take action that moves us forward one step at a time?

Like the Yin Qiao, this vessel begins in the region of the ankles, connects to the eyes and enters the brain. The Yin Qiao, which begins in the medial aspect of the ankles, gives us the internal alignment for the structure of the body-mind and the Yang Qiao, which begins in the lateral aspect of the ankles, governs the large muscle groups and joints that allow us to move through space. The Yin Qiao gives us insight for self-illumination and the Yang Qiao gives us a panoramic view of the world around us. Both vessels enter the brain and therefore have a strengthened relationship to the Sea of Marrow. The Yin Qiao treats accumulation in the abdomen and the Yang Qiao treats accumulation in the head.

YANG QIAO AND LOCOMOTION

As an offspring of the Du Mai, the Yang Qiao is responsible for bringing the yang qi of the Du Mai into the musculoskeletal system and head in order to provide balance and the ability to move with ease. A healthy Yang Qiao maintains the integrity of the three bony cavities of the body: the pelvis, the ribcage and the skull. This integrity is what allows us to walk upright. An upright posture has its benefits and is perhaps the key structural difference between humans and other mammals. The ability to walk upright frees up the arms and shoulders (SI-10, LI-15) giving both access to and mastery of the world around us that other mammals lack. It also changes the priority of our senses, making vision our most important sense. Most mammals use smell as their primary sense, but standing upright takes our nose away from the ground, shifting the focus to the eyes (UB-1).

The Yang Qiao governs how much yang qi is supplied to the superficial tissues. When the Yang Qiao is healthy and its circulation is free then we are comfortable in our movement. We can easily act or react appropriately and our body-mind connection is ready to respond to whatever is happening in the moment. This is about being present to what is. We are available to the present moment in a mindful way. When there is integrity in the Yang Qiao we are not thinking about something else or wishing we were some other place. Freedom in the Yang Qiao gives us the capacity to be fully present to what is occurring in our lives as it is occurring. If there is resistance in our structure or armoring in the soft tissues of the body, the Yang Qiao is in a state of excess. This excess causes pain, which can prevent us from being present in the moment.

YANG QIAO AND YANG WEI

The Yang Qiao and the Yang Wei have two very important intersection points where the arms and legs meet the torso at the shoulders and the hips. The Yang Wei governs how we deal with the future based on the past. When there is pathology in the Yang Wei people tend to get "stuck," unable to move forward due to fear or unresolved feelings. Those feelings and the stuck-ness associated with those feelings are transmitted to the Yang Qiao. When this occurs, the structure becomes tense and armored, bracing for a repeat of previous experiences, which then affects our ability to move freely and be present in the moment. If we were physically abused as a child or if we were bullied when we were in school then we develop a physiological response to the emotions of being attacked. We become armored against the abuse and we carry that tension into the present moment, continuously bracing ourselves for the next attack. It is interesting to note that there does not even need to be physical contact for this pattern to occur. A serious threat of physical contact is enough to start the pattern of tension that leads to the anticipation of pain and injury. It is almost impossible to be present in the moment when you are constantly waiting for the next attack.

Let's say as children we were told to "mind our own business." Then every time we tried to engage the world around us or participate in what was happening in the moment we were told to go away or threatened with some punishment. Eventually we respond to this indoctrination in one of two ways. We can either respond to these threats by creating tension in the Yang Qiao, which will then make us reluctant to engage for obvious self-preservation reasons, or we can rebel against the threat and thrust ourselves into the moment regardless of the consequences. Either option will cause tension in the Yang Qiao, which impedes our ability to move freely and easily in the world.

YANG QIAO AND HOLDING BACK

The withdrawal response creates a tremendous amount of tension from holding back. This can be seen in how patients hold themselves or in how they move as if they are waiting for the next shoe to drop or the next threat to occur. This holding can, over time, create an internal tension that causes these patients to implode. We frequently hear news stories where some seemingly nice, quiet, even-tempered person finally loses it and does something horrendously violent. These people have been holding that fear, anger and resentment contained in the tissues of the Yang Qiao until they cannot hold it anymore. People with this type of tension are prone to physiological implosions like high blood pressure, migraines, strokes and seizures. This constraint typically starts slowly with early warning symptoms like joint pain or rebellious qi symptoms like gastroesophageal reflux disease (GERD), belching or allergies. If we ignore the early warnings or attempts to communicate, or if we cannot find a way to release this tension then the Yang Qiao will find a way to release it for us.

YANG QIAO AND REBELLION

The other response to a childhood of having our freedom constrained is rebellion. We want things to be different; we want to change the world and those who would hold us back. So, we actively engage the world pushing beyond the fear of the consequences of childhood misbehavior. This sometimes comes in the form of overt or radical activism. We cannot accept the world the way it is and we will do whatever we can to change it. Somehow we think if we can do this then we will be alright, that our freedom will be restored and we will finally be the people we were meant to be. This driving force to fix the world creates tension in the Yang Qiao and we are sure that the tension will be relieved when we have completed our task of making the world right again.

This is quite different from the Yin Qiao approach of maintaining a relationship to the world. When the Yin Qiao is imbalanced and this imbalance results in an awareness that the world is not a happy place, the Yin Qiao pushes us towards changing ourselves in order to change the world. This is the Gandhi approach of "be the change you want to see in the world" or the "man in the mirror" approach to saving the world. In the Yang Qiao pathology everything is focused externally. The Yang Qiao has us constantly pushing against the world, which is both painful and exhausting. Sometimes the exhaustion that comes from this constant firing of the muscles leads us to feel defeated in the face of the seemingly insurmountable job of changing the world, and withdrawal then may seem like the best choice. This causes the pathology of the Yin Qiao to emerge, leading to symptoms like depression and chronic fatigue.

More often than not the rebellion can linger for years, surrounding us with conflict. When we are in this state, we are extroversion unchecked. We are like runaway freight trains unable to slow down enough to listen to what others have to say. We are unable to slow down enough to take on fuel or recharge. We are unable to slow down enough to see the futility of our actions. Our eyes are focused on the bigger goal of getting to the end of the line. With this big-picture vision we often miss the small details we would see if we were present to the moment. This in turn makes the conflict and tension worse because others are left to deal with the details and pick up what we miss. Runaway freight trains leave a mess on the tracks.

YANG QIAO AND CHRONIC PAIN

Chronic pain in the Yang Qiao, especially in the head, neck, shoulders, hips and low back, is a pretty good indicator that we are unable to be present in the moment. Few people understand that in order to be present in the moment we must learn to embrace the pain and accept the reality of the present. We need to make friends with it before we can move forward. Most of us look at pain as a distraction or an inconvenience that is making the pursuit of our goals more challenging. The pain however is actually trying to tell us to slow down. It is trying to get us to shift the balance from the extreme extroversion of the Yang Qiao more towards the introspection of the Yin Qiao. Our spirits use the pain to get us to find a way to bring balance between the Yin and Yang Qiao. If there is balance, there is alignment. If there is alignment, there is freedom. The spirit wants to be free.

YANG QIAO AND JUDGMENT

If your patient has an excess in the Yang Qiao, one of the least productive things you can do is tell them to relax. First of all, many of them think they are already relaxed and even if they don't, telling them to relax will feel like judgment to them. Once they feel judged by you then you become part of the world they are trying to change. They will rebel or withdraw and you will lose the opportunity to support them in their desire for change.

These patients want to be more relaxed; they want to be free. They believe the way to achieve that is to keep going. They want to keep pushing at the world until it gives in and changes. They believe they will relax when they are done. In patients like this you can try to free up the intersections between the Yang Wei and the Yang Qiao (SI-10 and GB-29). This will allow patients the opportunity to disengage or detach from their history or their anticipated future. It leaves them more of a chance to focus on the here and now.

YANG QIAO PATHWAY

The pathway of the Yang Qiao begins at the master point UB-62 and intersects with UB-61 and UB-59 in the area around the lateral malleolus. From here it rises up the lateral aspect of the leg, connecting with the Yang Wei at GB-29 continuing up the flank to the shoulder at SI-10, LI-15 and LI-16. From here it rises along the side of the neck to St-4, St-3 and St-1 on the face where it intersects with the Yin Qiao at UB-1. The pathway then enters the brain and emerges at GB-20, once again connecting it to the Yin Qiao. This pathway allows us to maintain an upright posture, see the world around us, take a stand and move out into the world from that stance.

Common conditions treated by the Yang Qiao

- Headaches, especially those related to excess (yang rising, liver fire, exterior wind and blood stasis).
- Mental problems: mania, agitation and insomnia
- Eye problems (tendency for the eyes to stay open).
- Interior and exterior wind (day-time epilepsy).
- Musculoskeletal pain (neck, back, shoulders, hips and ankles).
- Wei syndrome with flaccidity in the lateral aspect of the leg with tightness in the medial aspect of the leg.
- Urinary problems due to excess conditions.
- Hemiplegia, especially following wind-stroke.

—— CHAPTER 8 ——

DAI MAI

aka: The Belt Vessel, The Girdle
Vessel, The Sea of Ming Men

In this way of viewing the 8 EV as the unfolding of jing,
the Dai Mai is the last of the extraordinary vessels. In the
beginning, the Chong Mai gives birth to the pure potential of
our curriculum in life. It supplies us with prenatal yin (Ren Mai)
and prenatal yang (Du Mai), which is then distributed over
time and in the moment by the Wei and Qiao vessels. So what is
left for the Dai Mai to do?

The Dai Mai has three very important functions:

- It integrates, regulates and harmonizes the functions of
  the other vessels.

- It provides a link between the prenatal nature of the 8
  EV and the postnatal function of the middle jiao (Spleen
  and Stomach).

- It provides an overflow system or repository for unresolved
  emotions or trauma that affect the will to live (Jing).

There are two pathways of the Dai Mai: one that is more
prenatal in nature that can be used to support and consolidate
and one that is more postnatal in nature that can be used to
drain or detoxify.

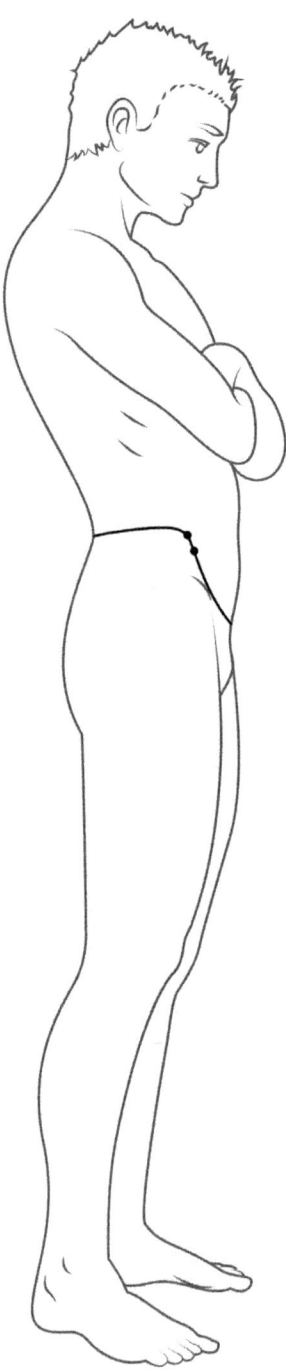

Figure 8.1: Dai Mai

Prenatal Dai: Du-4, UB-23, UB-52, GB-26, Sp-15, St-25, Ki-16, Ren-8

This pathway wraps around the middle like a belt, extending from the Kidney divergent meridian at Du-4 and following the waistline all of the way around the body to Ren-8. This vessel allows for integration to occur since all of the other vessels must pass through this belt.

Postnatal Dai: Lv-13, GB-26, GB-27, GB-28

This pathway also extends from the Kidney divergent meridian at Du-4, extends across the back and when it reaches the flank it follows the Gall Bladder pathway down into the lower jiao. The visual effect is more like a bucket or a basin than a belt. This aspect of the Dai Mai provides a region where trauma may be held in latency.

HARMONIZING AND INTEGRATING

The Dai Mai's horizontal trajectory allows it to come into contact with all of the other vertical pathways of the 8 EV. This pathway makes the Dai Mai particularly useful in the integration of the first ancestry (Chong, Du and Ren). The prenatal Dai Mai wraps completely around the midline of the body at the waist and each of the vessels in the first ancestry has a point on that pathway (Ki-16 on the Chong Mai, plus Du-4 and Ren-8).

You can think of this aspect of the Dai Mai as being somewhat like the lumbar support belt that one wears before doing some heavy lifting. The cinching (consolidating) of this belt supports the kidney region and in doing so gives support to the prenatal vessels.

SUPPORTING THE SPLEEN

The second function of providing a connection with the postnatal function of the Spleen is also related to its horizontal trajectory through the middle. But, this connection to the Spleen is primarily possible because of the heavy influence of the Gall Bladder channel in the Dai Mai pathway. Through its curious nature, the Gall Bladder provides a strong link between the constitution (yuan qi) and the postnatal function of the Spleen. Because the Gall Bladder is not a typical yang organ but rather an extraordinary fu, its function is strengthened by its connection to the 8 EV and yuan qi. It is, however, still part of the primary channel system that links it to postnatal function. It can therefore act as a bridge between the two. The Dai Mai can provide the transformative fire of Ming Men (Kidney yang) through the Gall Bladder to the Spleen to support the healthy functions of transformation and transportation (T & T). If the Dai Mai is weak and needs consolidating then the fire of Ming Men and Kidney yang will also be weak and unable to support digestive function. Strengthening the prenatal aspect of the Dai Mai will support the function of the Spleen. It can support transformation and transportation, strengthening the ability of the patient to digest both food and life. It can also insure the proper ascending and descending of qi out of the middle. Since the middle burner mediates the relationship between the upper and lower burners, strengthening this function helps to support the heart and kidney axis.

Typically, the Spleen generates dampness because it is too weak to transform and transport efficiently. If the Spleen generates enough dampness or if the Spleen dysfunction is not rectified then the yuan qi will be impeded. Turbid yin then rises up and affects the Sea of Marrow (brain) resulting in foggy-headedness, inability to focus or concentrate, poor memory, depression or dizziness. This obstruction of yin prevents the full expression of who we are. It affects our ability to take the outside world in. If our sensory orifices are veiled with yin then our perception of the world around us is clouded.

This is related to diet and lifestyle choices that do not support a well-functioning digestion. It is a postnatal issue, not constitutional in nature, but still we can treat this with the prenatal Dai Mai because it will support the function of the Spleen.

On occasion the Spleen is responding to a lifetime of poor choices and dietary improprieties. This might include things like smoking or drinking excessively. Under these circumstances the Spleen generates dampness as a form of self-preservation, usually in response to heat caused by poor lifestyle choices. We are using water to put out the fire. When we see dampness accumulating we must be careful to remove the dampness only when the fire that is evoking the dampness is addressed. If we take the dampness away before dealing with the fire, the fire will flare up. If we suspect that the dampness is a response to heat we can combine our Dai Mai (GB-41) treatment with the Yang Wei (SJ-5). One of the functions of the Yang Wei is to vent heat to the surface so that the Spleen/Dai Mai has no need to generate the dampness.

UNRESOLVED ISSUES THREATENING JING

Its third function is to act as a reservoir or receptacle for unresolved issues that threaten jing. We need only to look at the connection between the Dai Mai and the function of the lower jiao to understand this. The postnatal pathway of the Dai Mai (Lv-13, GB-26, GB-27, GB-28) creates a bucket or basin in the pelvic region that absorbs excesses from the postnatal system. These excesses represent postnatal experiences that cannot be effectively transformed and released. It may be unwanted memories of painful events, deeply held emotions or beliefs that are detrimental to our ability to pursue our purpose. It may also be trauma that we have experienced earlier in our lives that we did not have the capacity or resources to deal with at the time the trauma was occurring.

These experiences affect our will to live and so we store them down into the Dai Mai as far away from the heart as we can get and then we accumulate dampness in order to weigh down the feelings associated with those traumatic events and diminish our access to them. It's a little like taking the memories and feelings of the worst day of your life (a day that made you feel as though you wanted to die) and putting those feelings into a box, then putting the box down in a dark corner of the basement under a bunch of other boxes and then flooding the basement. After a while you notice the flooding because things are starting to leak but you have forgotten about the box in the dark corner.

This is a step beyond the self-preservation mechanism of creating latency. We are not looking to hold something at bay until we can gather the resources, support or wisdom to handle it later. We are looking to forget it ever existed. This is suppression and the cost of this suppression is high, as is the burden of the fluids that maintain it. This suppression dampens the fire of Ming Men and impedes the motive force of yang, which means we will have greater difficulty moving forward in life. We will have trouble transforming. We will feel heavy, tired and lethargic. We will feel stuck. This is like walking through life in waist-deep water. Every step is slow, laborious and typically ineffective in getting us where we really want to go. It is one thing to jump into a swimming pool and walk from side to side in order to get a little exercise; it is another to live every moment of your day walking through waist deep water. Imagine how exhausted you would feel. If every movement feels so effortful, pretty soon you might stop trying. You might begin to feel defeated. You may begin to lose your will.

DAI MAI AND WEIGHT GAIN

Although some people with Dai Mai issues carry extra weight around their middle as a visible sign of accumulation, that is not always the case. People who are not overweight can also have Dai Mai imbalances. Obstruction of the Dai Mai may present as low back pain, prostatitis, painful periods due to fibroids or cysts, impotence, painful intercourse and infertility. Instead of the extra weight there are painful physical signs of obstruction and accumulation in the lower burner. Their accumulation is internal and less visible or obvious but it still requires resources to maintain and it may also come about as a way of hiding or suppressing something.

At some point the accumulation in the Dai Mai may start to spill over and cause leakage. The dampness used to support the suppression places a burden on the jing which is trying hard to maintain the latency. This burden makes it difficult to contain in the lower burner and people develop diarrhea, frequent urination, vaginal discharge, edema and premature ejaculation. At some point the patient just cannot maintain the holding function in the lower burner and the dampness they have created to maintain the latency starts to leak. This is the body's way of saying: "I just can't hold onto to this anymore. I simply do not have the resources to keep this trauma, emotion or belief hidden away from consciousness anymore. You need to deal with this as soon as possible."

CONSOLIDATION OR RELEASE

When we treat the Dai Mai we must take the time to be certain that the patient has the courage and the resources to let go of that which no longer serves. It is important to know if they have the necessary support to lay down the burden they have been carrying, sometimes for years. Patients may be aware that they need to let go of something in order to move on but this can present certain challenges because these patients have suppressed trauma and in doing so they may not even be aware of why they are suffering. Also, the entrenchment caused by the dampness can make some of these patients quite stubborn or reluctant to do what needs to be done in order to let go. They often form deep resentments that make letting go of their past challenging. It may be wise to determine if these patients need to have their prenatal Dai Mai consolidated before draining the damp away. By consolidating first, we can stop the loss of qi and jing caused by the leakage. This gives the patient some time to recover from the loss of resources. It gives them some time to prepare to finally let go of that which no longer serves them in the pursuit of their destiny.

When patients are ready to have the Dai Mai drained the result can be a presence of mind and clarity of thought that the patient has not experienced in a long while. The removal of the dampness gives patients the room to breathe and feel without the obstruction or stuckness caused by the dampness. Freeing up the Dai Mai also makes more room for new latency to be created when needed. This is an important self-preservation mechanism. It is important to have a little room in the Dai Mai for when patients are challenged by life's overwhelming experiences.

SAN JIAO AND DAI MAI

The dampness in the Dai Mai may sometimes be more constitutional than postnatal. In the postnatal aspect we have created the dampness to reduce heat or to distance us from trauma and overwhelming experiences. There are times, however, when the dampness may accumulate in response to conflict created within our sense of ourselves. During the birth process the San Jiao/Triple Burner disseminates yuan qi to the zang organs. This is not necessarily a symmetrical process. Life is not fair nor equal and neither is the dissemination of yuan qi. The unevenness of this dissemination accounts not only for our constitutional strengths and weakness but also for our individuality. This is part of what makes each of us unique. Some babies are born calm and peaceful; others are quick to explore and engage the world around them. Some are easy to laugh and some are discontented or uncomfortable from the beginning. We can see very early on the budding of a distinct personality. If we cannot come to some level of self-acceptance of that which makes us unique, if we do not like aspects of ourselves, then the Dai Mai will generate dampness to soften those aspects of our personality that cause us pain. This dampness holds back the expression of those aspects of self that we find disconcerting. Unfortunately, in doing this it also slows or blocks the further dissemination of yuan qi to the zang organs. Once again the dampness weighs us down and stops us from moving forward.

This dampening of personality traits is not treated with the postnatal Dai Mai but rather with the pathway of the prenatal Dai Mai, which engages the function of Kidney yang for transformation. Lv-13 can be a useful addition to this type of treatment, as it is the influential point of the zang organs and it is on the pathway of the Dai Mai. When we include this point it allows the yuan qi to be disseminated more freely to the zang organs. This in turn may ease the suffering that one experiences from not liking aspects of ourselves.

DAI MAI AND GENTLE DRAINAGE

It is very important to remember that the dampness of the Dai Mai is not simply a postnatal pathology. It is a survival strategy. The dampness in the Dai Mai occurs when there is a threat to jing. If you are unsure of that threat then perhaps it is best to treat the Spleen first. If treating the Spleen does not work then you can consider the Dai Mai as the impediment to clearing the dampness.

If you use the Dai Mai without respect for the self-preservation aspect you will leave your patient feeling vulnerable. For some, the experience of vulnerability is just the thing they need to face their past. Perhaps those patients are able to deal with the vulnerability because they now have a better support system. Perhaps they have gained wisdom and capacity with age. Whatever the reason, they are now prepared to be a little uncomfortable in order to let go and move on.

For others, that vulnerability is like being retraumatized. As the Dai Mai is opened and the veil of dampness is drained away, all of those uncomfortable feelings return. The feelings may be accompanied by recall in the form of flashbacks or nightmares. They may surface in confusing or disorienting ways. This can once again be overwhelming to the patient. They may feel as though they are not ready or prepared to deal with this re-surfacing.

The most important tenet of all medicine is: "first do no harm." So if we decide to drain the Dai Mai we must try to find a way to do this as gently as possible. I frequently combine the Ren Mai (Lu-7) with my Dai Mai treatments (GB-41). The Ren Mai as the Sea of Yin can be used to drain dampness but it is also one of the most important vessels for establishing a connection to self and supporting self-love. As the vessel of closure, the Ren Mai helps us to move on after trauma and as the vessel of containment it may minimize the loss of vital substances in the draining process. In my practice, this particular combination has been proven to be both compassionate and effective in draining away the dampness that is inhibiting the fullest expression of who were are.

DAI MAI AND DETOXIFICATION

If you have a patient who is robust in constitution and is experiencing excess symptoms related to the Dai Mai then you may need to begin the 8 EV journey by clearing the Dai Mai first. Draining the Dai Mai makes room for the rest of the process to emerge. You are detoxifying the body—removing the excess or obstructions that may be preventing the patient from experiencing anything else in their bodies. The world today can be a pretty toxic environment and in order to survive that toxicity the body kicks into self-preservation mode and attempts first to eliminate those toxins. If it is unable to eliminate them all, it will find a safer place to hold those toxins. Draining the Dai Mai can be useful in removing those toxins that are held in latency deep in the lower jiao. Starting with the Dai Mai can actually also make it easier for the practitioner to see what needs to be balanced or perhaps allow the root pattern to emerge. Once the toxicity is removed the curriculum can begin to present itself.

THE DAI MAI AND DEEPLY HELD BELIEFS

The Dai Mai is an incredibly important vessel for self-preservation but it can also be the impediment to fulfilling our curriculum. It can provide us with support for the first ancestry and protect us from trauma that might overwhelm jing or it may be holding onto so much toxicity that we cannot move beyond the need to keep that toxicity in latency.

The Dai Mai may also be where some of our most deep and negative beliefs are being held. Early trauma may lead to us developing some negative beliefs about ourselves that are counterproductive to our growth and development. These beliefs often develop before we have the cognitive function to understand the context of the trauma we have experienced. For example, anyone suffering the violation of incest or sexual abuse in childhood has no way to create context for the betrayal of a trusted family member. They have no way of dealing with the mixed feelings that can arise from this abuse. If a family is destroyed when the abuse is revealed they may feel as if the loss of the family unit is all their fault, in the same way that children often feel that it is their fault that their parents are divorcing. Without the ability to create context for this trauma, fear, confusion, frustration and self-judgment, feelings of guilt or shame erupt. Those feelings begin to overwhelm the child so they get pushed down into the Dai Mai so that life can continue. The problem is that as life continues it is overshadowed by the negativity of those feelings. Future relationships are unconsciously framed in the suppressed memories and the feelings associated with earlier trauma. Failures and disappointments in life may become further justification for those deeply held beliefs. While patients are often unaware of these beliefs they are often living lives that are expressions of them. Helping those patients to find freedom from those deeply held and negative beliefs relieves them of a burden they may not even be aware they are carrying.

A healthy Dai Mai means that we have support in the middle to integrate and harmonize all of the vessels that flow vertically throughout the body. We have a tool for self-preservation and vessel that supports latency when jing is threatened. Its capacity for creating latency for survival is only supposed to be a stop-gap measure. It is designed to allow us some time to gather our resources and then eventually deal with that which has been repressed or suppressed. We cannot hold on to things that conflict with Self (yuan qi) forever. At some point we must let go. We must release those old hurts, those violations of our boundaries and those deeply held and critical beliefs. For if we cannot eventually release that which is stored in the Dai Mai, the conflict overwhelms Self. This means that we become something we were not meant to be or we die. In working constantly to maintain the latency we are directing our resources to that purpose. We cannot then use those resources to become more of who we are. That means there are less resources available with which to pursue meaning and purpose in life.

Common conditions treated by the Dai Mai

- Fullness around the middle.

- Dampness obstructing the lower burner (vaginal discharge, Shan disorders and urinary problems).

- Pain in the waist and lumbar regions.

- Headaches associated with Liver and Gall Bladder excess (heat, fire and damp-heat).

- Atrophy and leg qi: cold legs and feet (feels like sitting in cold water). Muscle pain in the legs.

- Gynecology and infertility conditions associated with damp obstruction, qi stagnation or failure to disseminate yuan qi from Ming Men.

- Prolapse due to Spleen qi sinking.

- Hip and groin pain.

PART 2

THE CLINICAL APPLICATION of the EIGHT EXTRAORDINARY VESSELS

—— CHAPTER 9 ——

INTENT VERSUS AGENDA

When a patient comes to us with acute onset low back pain because they improperly lifted a heavy box, we do what we can to relieve their pain. We may also counsel them on the proper ergonomics of lifting or we might recommend some exercises to strengthen the low back and core muscles of the abdomen. Our intent is to relieve the pain and insure that the patient is educated so they do not reinjure themselves.

It's all pretty straightforward and acupuncture is almost magical in its ability to deal with this type of pain. These patients come into our offices in agony. They often have difficulty getting onto the treatment table. After the treatment they rise up and say: "It's like a miracle; the pain is so much better. It's almost completely gone." When that happens, it is a good day in the clinic. We are reminded how amazing CM is and how accomplished we are as practitioners of this medicine. However, we can also fall into the trap of believing we are actually "fixing" someone. If we do fall into this trap, what happens to us when we meet a patient we cannot help? We may feel that we are a failure or we may blame the patient for not complying with our recommendations. That is the core issue of intent versus agenda.

What if we have a patient who has chronic low back pain and they have a flare up of that pain while they are moving some small boxes from their old home to their new home? With patients like these we have to be much clearer with our intent. If we accept that pain is a communication from the body then we must ponder what it is that the body is trying to communicate. Is the body trying to say: "You shouldn't be lifting anything with your bad back"? Is it trying to get the patient to recognize that there is an ongoing instability in the low back by speaking a little louder? "Hey! I've been trying to tell you for a long time now that we have a problem!" The pain may be the spirit's way of getting the patient to slow down a bit and become more aware of the emotions associated with the move. "We were really happy in this home and now we are moving to a place where everything is new and unknown." The pain may be related to an over-consumption of resources. "You have been working too hard lately and I need you to get more rest."

By the time most patients come to see us for acupuncture, they are suffering from pain or illness that is complex in nature and etiology. The current state of their being is seldom solely responsible for their suffering. The precipitating event is not usually the problem. So many times I have heard patients with back pain say things like: "I don't know what happened. I was perfectly fine and then all I did was bend over to pick up a pencil and WHAM, I couldn't move because of the pain." Bending over to pick up the pencil is obviously not the problem. Neither is the problem simply some structural imbalance that made the patient vulnerable to this type of injury. The body does not go on strike for lifting a pencil until it has tried many other ways to get the patient to pay attention. The real problem is a long-term disconnect from the communication that the spirit is trying to direct through the body.

With this type of complexity the question then becomes, how does one set an intention for treatment that addresses the patient's suffering within the larger context of listening and learning? How do we help the patient to develop the body awareness necessary so that they can hear the communication of the body before it has to scream to get their attention?

Do we focus on the physical pain? Do we focus on the weakness in structure? Do we focus on creating an awareness of how the patient came to this place of suffering?

If we focus solely on relieving the pain perhaps the patient will not get the message and continue to reinjure themselves. If we support the underlying weakness in structure or the lack of resources we are helping the patients to become stronger and maybe reducing the risk of reinjury but are we really addressing the source of the problem? Why are those resources depleted? What is it about how they are living their lives that creates this underlying weakness in structure? Do they have a history of injury or trauma? Are they living their lives severely out of balance with their resources?

Chapter 8 of the Ling Shu (Spiritual Pivot) begins with the Yellow Emperor asking physician Qibo about diseases caused by spiritual activities. Qibo answers the Yellow Emperor's question by laying out how man is created and how wisdom is developed and concludes by suggesting that the wise man lives in accordance with the natural order of things. Observing nature and living life in a natural and balanced way promotes health and longevity.

Although we are endowed with a certain innate knowingness, we must learn from the experiences we have in life. We have a prenatal gift of wisdom passed down from the previous generations but we must also learn from our postnatal experiences. We gain wisdom by living. Is there a way then that we can create an intent for our treatments that allows for those life lessons to be translated into wisdom?

After many years of treating patients with chronic pain or lingering illness or imbalance, I have seen that patients make the biggest adjustments to their lifestyles and the greatest improvements in their suffering if you address all three issues at the same time. The beauty of CM in general and the 8 EV specifically is that you can choose a vessel that will create an intent that acknowledges the physical pain, the structural weakness and the spiritual imbalance that inhibits the gathering of wisdom from experience.

To do this you must recognize that patients do not deliberately decide to go against the laws of nature. Most of us make bad choices in a moment of crisis because it seems like the simplest or best option available. Perhaps we make those choices because they have worked in the past. We may choose to override the body's communication because our fears or desires tell us to keep going. We may also develop habitual responses to life's challenges.

HABITUAL RESPONSES

Avoidance of conflict is an example of one of those behaviors that is often unconscious and habitual. If we are in the habit of avoiding conflict, we will often avoid those experiences that may be key in overcoming our current suffering. So how then do we develop that habitual response? Maybe in childhood we were faced with conflict and we withdrew as an act of self-preservation. Maybe we withdraw because we are frightened or confused and we need some time to consider the feelings stirred up by the conflict. Or perhaps we withdraw because we remember our parents saying: "Don't fight, just walk away." Although withdrawal may be prudent, when it becomes our coping style we may never get the opportunity to learn other ways to deal with conflict. We may not get the opportunity to gain in the wisdom that comes from experiencing conflict resolution. This coping style of avoidance is a limited approach and our spirit wants to expand our consciousness, not limit it. Avoidance works for immediate relief because it takes us away from the emotional charge of conflict but really that is no different than taking two aspirin for a headache. Yes, the headache will go away but then we continue to take aspirin every time we get a headache. At some point we will need to try to figure out why we are getting headaches. It is hoped we can manage to do that before the aspirin burns a hole in our stomach causing us a new focus for our suffering. If we avoid conflict as our coping style, that withdrawal may cause us to stagnate or accumulate pathological yin. The stagnation of yin then reinforces the withdrawal/avoidance. Simply removing the stagnation will not necessarily change the coping style and in fact in some cases the freedom in the circulation may lead to anxiety (internal conflict), which then evokes the coping mechanism in even stronger ways.

So how then can we create a treatment that has the intent of supporting the patient in their ability to face their fear and move forward? Can we create a treatment that will help the patient to understand that overcoming their suffering will only occur when they face the conflict? Can we create a treatment that supports the awareness that they have the capacity to engage their will, to move through conflict rather than running from it? Sometimes you just have to do the things you don't like to do for change to happen. Can we create a treatment that gives the patient enough courage and will to engage the conflict head on?

We set an intention that serves the patient in the healthiest possible way. One of the ways we know that our intention is as healthy as possible is by being sure that it lacks personal agenda. This begs the question: "What is the difference between intent and agenda?" Agenda is not only a list of things that need to be accomplished but also often includes a goal that is determined by some ideological understanding of the patient's suffering. That means that, if we have an agenda, we (practitioners) decide what is wrong, how it needs to be fixed and what it looks like when the problem is resolved.

An intent is a determination to do something but it is also the state of mind you inhabit when you do that thing. "I intend to create the best possible environment for the patient to embrace growth and healing," is not the same as "I know what is wrong and I intend to fix this patient." The first recognizes that it is the patient's choice and the second intention comes from a place of judgment or hubris. The second intent has a personal agenda. We know what our medicine can offer to our patients and we have been trained to make a diagnosis based on physiological signs and symptoms but we can never truly know the uniqueness of each of our patients. We can never truly know the meaning or purpose in another's life. It is not for us to judge whether suffering is productive or not. It is not for us to determine the how and when another will heal.

Here's a discussion that I frequently have with female patients who are approaching menopause:

Patient: My doctor wants me to go on hormones.

Me: Did he/she say why?

Patient: Yes, he/she says my estrogen is low and that is why I am having night sweats.

Me: Have you had your estrogen levels tested?

Patient: No, not yet, but I have all the signs.

Me: Did your doctor tell you that at your age your estrogen is supposed to be decreasing? Did he/she tell you that menopause serves a very important purpose for longevity?

Patient: Well…no. He/she just told me I would feel better if I went on the hormones.

The doctor has a well-meaning intent that has an agenda. The doctor knows that hormones will ease the physical suffering of this transition. There is a cost to be paid for the doctor's agenda. Supplementing with hormones will alter the nature of the transition and also may deny the patient the opportunity to gain the wisdom of this powerful time.

I am not suggesting that no one should use Hormone Replacement Therapy (HRT); sometimes the suffering is so great or arrives significantly earlier than normal, which may cause severe symptoms that distract from the learning opportunity. I am suggesting that the decision to use HRT should be accompanied by enough information and awareness that the patient knows both the benefits and challenges presented by making that choice. I am saying that it is up to the patient to decide how they will embrace that change and that it is not our place to judge their choices.

I feel obliged to inform my patients that there are cultures that make this transition easily, gracefully and without the support of hormonal supplementation. Women who live in societies that respect aging and support the unfolding of wisdom that comes with this transition often suffer less. What if we found a way to create a treatment intent that helped women understand the benefits that the menopause transition brings instead of just focusing on all the myriad symptoms that may or may not occur during this powerful time? What if we helped women to embrace aging and the potential wisdom that arises out of the change, whether or not they decide to use HRT?

We can create a treatment plan that gives the patient an opportunity to embrace this powerful transition. We can allow for the possibility that this transition will unfold in a way that is most appropriate for each patient. In this way the patient isn't avoiding the inevitable or ignoring the message of the body but is in fact embracing the change. When we can create an intent that includes the capacity to embrace change, the physical suffering typically decreases and our relationship to the suffering changes. We become less resistant and more available to the opportunity to gain in wisdom.

I believe that, as practitioners of an amazing system of medicine, it is incumbent upon us to develop clarity in our intent when helping our patients. I think we need to develop a level of compassionate detachment that embraces the idea that it is the patient who chooses to heal or not. That if we try to "fix" our patients we are, in a way, disempowering them and giving our own egos a little boost. When we look in a patient's eyes we must see the part of them that can never be injured and then support that. Of course we will address their symptoms and their suffering but not to the exclusion of their curriculum.

I am not saying that we should let our patient tells us what points to use or what herbs they need. We are well-educated medical professionals who know our medicine. But, even with all of our training, we can never really know what experiences a person needs to have in order to heal. I am suggesting that the patient takes the lead on determining the intent of the treatment. They tell us where they are in their healing process and what they feel they need to continue. We then turn that into the clearest intent of support for that patient's journey. It doesn't always look like we think it should. In my early days of practice I was referred a patient who in the section on chief complaint on her intake form listed anxiety, insomnia, addiction and wrinkles. She was young and quite beautiful and her skin was luminous. As was my habit, I asked her which of those four chief complaints was most important to her. The last thing I expected to hear was "wrinkles." In my arrogance and inexperience I decided that I was not a good fit for her. I felt as if she was so self-involved that her focus on her outside appearance was a distraction to what she really needed to work on. So, I referred her to a colleague who, by the way, treated her wrinkles, which surprise, surprise, surprise…had a beneficial effect on everything else. If I had been less wrapped up in my own sense of self-importance I would have been able to see that her self-image was intimately intertwined with her emotional instability. I would have seen that her suffering could be addressed by treating the symptom that to her was the most painful expression of that imbalance. All I could think about was how trivial it was that a patient this beautiful and youthful was worried about wrinkles. I wanted to project my values and my agenda onto her. In the end I was absolutely correct to refer her out. Not because she didn't understand what I could do for her but because I didn't understand her or her suffering. Her healing at the hands of another has been a powerful lesson for me.

These days I try hard to let my patients lead their healing process. I listen to what they believe is causing their suffering and I try to honor that. I do my job by providing them with information, exploring their history, seeking the imbalances and creating a treatment that addresses those imbalances. Then I leave it up to them how they will use that information and the treatment I provide. I am diligent about creating treatments with intent that empower the patient to take back their health in whatever way is best for them. The 8 EV help me to do that.

CHAPTER 10

CREATING A TREATMENT

There are a number of ways to create an 8 EV treatment. Perhaps as many ways as there are books on the 8 EV. So, let us begin by saying there is no one way to do this. I am going to suggest a basic structure that you might use to help you create an effective treatment. I recommend that you also read other practitioners' approaches and see what feel right to you.

When you first start to employ these treatments you may not understand the power of these vessels. You may feel inclined to use too many points or maybe you will want to add points that are not on the trajectory of the vessel in order to address a symptom your patient is experiencing. Here is a little advice that might help you to understand why that may not be the best or most effective idea.

First, most of us were trained to think about acupuncture through the lens of a zangfu (organ) diagnosis. We use the primary channel points to affect organ function. We use St-36 for symptoms in the abdomen especially those related to Spleen deficiency or damp accumulation; Ki-3, the source point of the kidney channel to tonify the kidneys. The 8 EV do not directly penetrate the organs. This is channel theory. The 8 EV are jing vessels that influence the vital substances and the curious organs. If you add points that are not on the trajectory of the vessel you may be sending mixed messages and you will be unable to understand fully the effect of that vessel. Especially in the beginning, you might just try to trust the vessel to do its job.

You can treat digestion through the Ren Mai and you can also treat dampness, which is a yin pathogen, with the Ren Mai (Sea of Yin) so there is often no need to add St-36 to support the postnatal function.

PROCESSING INFORMATION

I am a big fan of the "less is more" theory. Each needle is a piece of information that needs to be processed by your patient. If your patient actually needs an 8 EV treatment then it is highly likely that their capacity to process information or experience is already compromised. Yuan qi (source qi) is the qi of function and jing is its densest expression. So if you are treating yuan qi then function is compromised. If you can provide the patient with just a little information that is concise and has a clear intent or context then the patient may be better able to receive and respond to that information.

Keeping things simple and clear is also the best way to learn from the treatments you create. If you write a formula that has four to six individual herbs in it you will find it much easier to understand the effect of that formula than a formula with 15 herbs in it.

To that end, I recommend that you start with one vessel at a time or, if you need to combine them, no more than two at a time. This will allow you to determine more easily the effect of your treatment. You do not need to use them in the typical nuclear pairing. The Ren Mai does not need to be combined with the Yin Qiao. You can pair the Yin Qiao with the Yang Qiao or the Ren Mai can be combined with the Dai Mai. This should only be done if you understand the functions of each vessel and where their functions overlap.

If you have trouble determining which vessel you want to use, Jeffrey Yuen recommends beginning with the Chong or Dai. The Chong can help the patient to build the resources necessary to deal with the pathology and the Dai's detoxifying function can be used to clear a pathway for removal of the pathology. Either of these vessels can help to illuminate the real problem, making it easier to determine which vessel is next to be treated. Many of my patients have psycho-emotional disorders related to early or severe trauma so for me starting with the Dai can be a little risky. It can be a little like opening Pandora's Box. You cannot know for sure what will happen when you open the box and allow those old suppressed memories and traumas to surface. However, if you have a patient who has a robust constitution and needs support for detoxification then the Dai Mai is an excellent way to do that.

With that advice in mind, here is the approach I recommend: Choose a vessel. Start first with the master point of the vessel you want to open. You can think of the master point like a key that unlocks the door to the vessel, especially when needled with deeper intent and the appropriate technique. If you want to open the Chong Mai, the first point in is Sp-4. It is interesting to note that in some of the classical texts there are discussions of the 8 EV without the master points. The master points were added much later. This implies that you could in effect do 8 EV treatments without them, using only the points on the pathway. Ritual strengthens intent, so using the master point and establishing it as the key by inserting it first can create a stronger and clearer intent. Since the master points are also points on the primary channels, to be clear about your intent you will need to add points on the trajectory of the vessel you have chosen. Choose the points that will treat your patient's chief complaint and also choose points that are in alignment with your intent. For instance, in a Du Mai treatment, after first inserting SI-3, you might choose Du-4 for a chief complaint of chronic low back pain. You might also choose Du-14 and Du-20 to support the spinal axis and help the patient to stand upright with courage and will. If there is emotional constraint either triggering or aggravating the back pain you might want to use Du-9 to open the diaphragm and release the constraint in the chest.

You may then decide whether or not to add the couple point to your treatment. You can do a very effective Chong Mai treatment for instance, without the couple point Pc-6. But if your patient has a sense of internal urgency, anxiety or tension in the chest than you might want to include it in your treatment. In this way you are using some of the resources of the Yin Wei to support the function of the Chong Mai.

Every now and then you will run into a situation where two vessels seem to have equal importance in the pathology of your patient. For instance you may find it difficult to decide between the Du and the Ren and you will want to do both. In that case, you might use both master points and points along the trajectory of both vessels. Whatever vessel you deem to have the primary pathology might then be supported by using a greater number of points on the trajectory of that vessel.

FREQUENCY OF TREATMENTS

I typically treat patients no more than once a week if I am using the 8 EV. I like to have time for the treatment to unfold and new awareness to emerge. Chinese Medicine like Chinese philosophy values numbers. There is something magical about treating a patient every seven days with the 8 EV. The 8 EV govern the seven/eight-year cycles of jing. I like the resonance. Many of my patients need more time than seven days for the treatments to evolve so they come less often. I have patients I see every two or even three weeks and some who come for a treatment and don't return until they are ready for the next thing. These treatments don't seem to lose their effect if you delay the next treatment but they can cause discomfort if you treat too often. You can only treat at a pace that is consistent with the patient's capacity for consciousness. If you have patients who are used to being treated twice a week then by all means, treat them. I recommend that only one of those treatments be an 8 EV.

YIN, YANG AND SIDES OF THE BODY

Right? Left? Yin? Yang? Which side do you needle the master point on? Here are some thoughts on that. Traditionally, we say that the right side of the body is yin and the left is yang but from a prenatal perspective the opposite is true. The right is yang and the left is yin. You would think that simplifies everything but it doesn't because the first ancestry is prenatal and the second and third ancestries are considered postnatal. To complicate matters even more, the Chong Mai and the Dai Mai have both pre and postnatal expressions. Here's what that looks like:

- **Prenatal Chong**: left in females, right in males.

- **Postnatal Chong**: right in females, left in males.

- **Ren Mai** is the prenatal source of yin so it is needled on the left in both males and females.

- **Du Mai** is the prenatal source of yang so it is needled on the right in both males and females.

- **Wei and Qiao** vessels are postnatal, so right in females and left in males.

- **Prenatal Dai**: left in females, right in males.

- **Postnatal Dai**: right in females, left in males.

Now far be it from me to cause any more confusion at the moment that you might think you have a rule that you can follow. The 8 EV have pulses associated with them. If you happen to be using pulse confirmation then you can needle the master point on the side that the 8 EV pulse is confirmed. If you feel a Ren Mai pulse on the right then you needle Lu-7 on the right. You are such a rule-breaker! If the 8 EV pulse is palpable bilaterally then guess what... You can needle the master points bilaterally! It's all about guidelines, not rules and protocols. Sometimes I will even needle the master point on the side that is affected physiologically. For instance, if I am doing a Yang Qiao treatment for musculoskeletal problems like neck pain then I might needle UB-62 on the side that has the worst pain.

What I find is that unilateral use of the master point or unilateral use of the trajectory points seems to produce a stronger result. It seems to create more movement. My understanding of that is based on the theory that "nature abhors a vacuum." If you leave one side open the qi in the channel will move towards the empty space. On the other hand, bilateral treatment seems to create more balance and containment and therefore seems to be a little gentler. You get to decide what will serve your patient best. I think it is important to add that Li Zhi Shen is said to have preferred the unilateral approach, suggesting that it is more respectful. One only needs a single key to open a lock. So I try to respect the master when I can but sometimes I just feel the need to rebel against convention.

A word about needle technique. When you needle an acupuncture point and you achieve a qi sensation that means you have connected with ying qi. In an 8 EV treatment you want to access the qi more deeply at the level of yuan qi. This can be done by three methods: vibrating, shaking or listening. Descriptions of these techniques can be found in Ann Cecil-Sterman's book, *Advanced Acupuncture, A Clinic Manual.* I would also suggest that you can direct your intent deeper into the system with the idea that your insertion should create deep waves that cause the jing to respond. Your patients will feel the difference. You do not need to learn these needle techniques before you do 8 EV treatments. This is another ritual that deepens the intent. Needle technique is important but it is not the only ritual that makes the treatment effective.

ADDITIONAL POINTS

Even though I have recommended that you keep things simple in the beginning, I know that some of you will feel strongly about adding additional points. What follows is an explanation of which classifications of points will be more aligned with your treatment. You will want to stay away from any points that will distract from your intent or the intent of the vessel you have chosen.

Any point that has a relationship to yuan qi can be added without causing a distraction. That includes: Front-mu, Back-shu, He-sea, Influential, San Jiao (Triple Burner), Divergent confluent points, Luo, Source, Kidney, Ren and Du points.

Front-mu and **Back-shu** points regulate organ function and function is a yuan qi issue. The Back-shu points are on the inner line of the Urinary Bladder channel and as such are thought to be an extension of the Du Mai (source yang).

He-sea points have the deepest impact of the five transporting points. Like a large river flowing into the sea they are said to move inward to the depths.

Influential points, sometimes called the Gathering (hui) points, have an influence on specific tissues. Many of these tissues are associated with the curious organs. The qi is said to gather or concentrate here affecting the function of those tissues. The curious organs are influenced by the 8 EV.

San Jiao (Triple Heater) points may be added because the San Jiao is the avenue of yuan qi. It is said to disseminate yuan qi in all three burners, allowing the yuan qi to penetrate the organs.

The **Divergent confluent points,** sometimes called the "upper and lower meeting points," can also be used, because it is the function of the Divergent system to strengthen the relationship between yuan qi and wei qi. The lower meeting points diverge from the primary channel into the level of yuan qi and the upper meeting points allow for the yuan qi to surface at the level of wei qi in the region of the head and neck.

Luo points connect to source points and **source points** are the points on the channel where yuan qi is disseminated.

The **Kidney points** can also be used, since the kidneys store jing. They are the source vessels of the primary channel system.

You can also add **Ren** or **Du** points to any other 8 EV treatment. As the vessels of yuan yin and yuan yang they have a deep and profound relationship to yuan qi.

Once again I recommend keeping it simple. If you feel the need to add any of these points to your treatment, try to insure that you are not overwhelming the intent of the vessel you have chosen or overwhelming the patient with too much information.

These vessels are archetypal in nature. They each have a specific resonance or personality if you will. The more you work with them the more you will come to understand their beauty, simplicity and elegance.

What follows are some sample treatments based on imaginary patients. This is an exercise in helping you to understand the decisions you might make in order to create a treatment. There is a sample treatment for each of the vessels and two for the Dai Mai. These are not protocols. They are approaches to creating an opportunity for the patient to change their relationship to their suffering. I will do my best to explain why I chose the points I did and also why you may want to use different or additional points.

CHONG MAI

Let's imagine that your patient has a history of chronic digestive problems with difficulty assimilating nutrients. In the primary channel system this is most likely related to a deficient spleen. This patient may be suffering from depression or excessive worrying or perhaps they are couch potatoes who are unable to assimilate life. This lack of transformation and transportation often causes problems with blood, including a failure to generate blood or blood stasis. There may even be a failure to hold blood in the vessels, causing easy bruising or heavier menses.

We might in this instance think about the fifth trajectory of the Chong Mai. The fifth trajectory supports the relationship between the Sea of Nutrition and the Sea of Blood to insure that adequate assimilation occurs.

The treatment might look something like this:

- **Sp-4**: right in females, left in males (this is for postnatal function).

Then we might choose from the following points on the fifth trajectory:

- St-30, St-36, St-37, St-39, St-42, Lv-1, Sp-1.

- **Sea of Nutrition points**: St-30 and St-36 to strengthen the ability to assimilate food and life.

- **Sea of Blood points**: St-37 and St-39 to generate enough blood to create ballast for the emotional experience. In supporting the blood we are supporting the patient's ability to bring context to their memories and mediate their emotions.

- **St-42** is the source point of the stomach and it supports the ascending of clear yang.

- **Lv-1** can be used for blood stasis caused by the lack of assimilation (transportation and transformation).

- **Sp-1** for disturbances in the shen or bleeding problems caused by the lack of assimilation.

- If, for instance, part of the problem is the liver invading the spleen then you might do both of the jing-well points. If you want to add points you might consider the source points of the liver, spleen or kidney.

REN MAI

A 38-year-old male patient has anxiety. The anxiety has been something he has battled for as long as he can remember. He remembers being very fearful as a child even though his mom was always there trying to protect him. He is very close to his mom. He also has a lot of frustrations in his life. He does not deal well with failure. He is a picky eater. His tongue is dusky and his pulse is long and wiry in the middle level, especially on his left (prenatal yin). His pathological relationship with his mother and food leads us to the Ren Mai.

- **Lu-7** on the left (prenatal yin) opens the Ren Mai.

- **Ki-6** on the right is the coupled point of the Ren Mai and will provide the patient with the sensation of being more grounded and it will also help illuminate the reasons for the anxiety.

- **Ren-15** threaded down towards **Ren-14.** Ren-15 and Ren-14 calm the shen and reduce anxiety but when you connect the two of them together by threading you use one less needle to restore the relationship between the heart and kidney. You direct the fire back down to where it belongs. You could also palpate the Ren Mai for tender or empty points and add what you thought was needed or you could leave the focus on the heart at Ren-15 and Ren-14.

- If there is heat along the anxiety you could add **LI-11**. LI-11 may be considered the he-sea point of the 8 EV. This point has a broad band effect that is similar to the functions of the 8 EV. It can eliminate all kinds of heat at any level of the body.

- If the heat is coming from an imbalance in the relationship between the heart and kidney then you might consider **Ki-2** as it is on the trajectory of the coupled vessel (Yin Qiao).

- If the patient has obvious symptoms of qi stagnation you might consider adding either **Lv-14** to regulate the function of the liver or **Ren-6** to circulate the qi in the abdomen. If there is constraint in the chest causing pain you might consider using **Ren-17**.

DU MAI

Your patient is a 32-year-old female patient who has a chief complaint of depression. The depression is characterized by apathy and a lack of will. She has difficulty getting out of bed in the morning and would probably stay in bed all day long if it weren't for the overwhelming need to evacuate her bowels. Her stool is loose, watery and has undigested food. She has lost her passion for life and does not want to engage the world anymore because she feels as if she never wins. Her tongue is pale, swollen and wet and her pulse is floating, large and weak. Her yang is outward floating and the fire of Ming Men is waning. The loss of motive force associated with yang deficiency leads us to the Du Mai.

- **SI-3** on the right (prenatal yang is right).

- Then one might add any point on the Du Mai but using **Du-4, Du-14** and **Du-20** engages the motive force of yang and gets the patient upright and moving.

- You would need to decide whether to use **UB-62,** the couple point, with this treatment. It may indeed be helpful here for a couple of reasons: the Yang Qiao is the vessel of locomotion and it also enters the brain and could impact the brain chemistry that is dysregulated with the depression. If you do decide to add it use it on the left, contralateral to SI-3.

- Another point you might consider in a treatment like this is **UB-52**; the outer shu of the kidneys engages the will.

YIN WEI

A 33-year-old female patient is suffering from a broken heart. She broke up with her boyfriend last week and she can't sleep. She has had several broken relationships since she was 16 years old. She says she cannot forget her first love who broke her heart when he went off to college and left her behind. She feels a deep dull pain in her chest and abdomen as she aches for the way things used to be. In all of her relationships something has always been missing. No matter how hard she tries she just can't find "the one."

This patient is stuck in a fantasy world, longing for a past that no longer exists. This is a Yin Wei disorder.

- I might use **Pc-6** and **Lv-3** in an "infinity loop" meaning I might start with Pc-6 on the right then do Lv-3 on the left, Lv-3 on the right and finish with Pc-6 on the left. This particular "figure 8" pattern is sometimes called the "inner gates." It creates a similar type of movement to the "four gates" (LI-4 and Lv-3). When you use Pc-6 instead of LI-4 it will address the deep internal stagnation that is associated with emotional constraint. You begin with the Pc-6 because this will be a Yin Wei treatment for the broken heart.

- **Lv-14** releases the qi stagnation that is obstructing the diaphragm and chest but it also serves another purpose. As the last point on the ying qi cycle it represents endings and what follows endings is new beginnings. So this point can help to instill a sense of hope that things can change. Its name, Cycle Gate, implies that life cycles on. What follows sundown is sunrise, a new day, a new start.

- **Sp-15** supports the spleen's function of transformation and transportation. It helps patients to digest life's experiences and make some sense of them. This allows us to learn from that experience and carry that knowledge into the next experience.

- **Ki-9** is the xi-cleft point of the Yin Wei so it can be said to remove blockages from the interior including old memories or old pains that hold us hostage in the past.

That is a complete treatment; it needs nothing else to create a powerful intent. However, there may be reasons to add more points or perhaps different points:

- One could add either **Ren-22** or **Ren-23** if the patient was having difficulty speaking their truth or difficulty swallowing a distasteful or uncomfortable experience.

- If the patient is an emotional eater or the heartbreak is causing them to have food cravings then you might consider using **Sp-16** instead of Sp-15.

YANG WEI

Let's say you have a male patient who is depressed and stuck in a bit of a mid-life crisis. He is not dealing with physical limitations that sometimes occur with aging. He may have started with an injury to his shoulder at the gym and the reality of the recovery time and care needed to reintroduce physical activity may have caused some frustration. So now let's say he has some recurring sensitivity in the shoulder, which is giving him some neck problems upon rotation of the head and his hips have become achy, especially the one on the opposite side of the shoulder pain. His frustration at not being able to maintain his exercise regime or having joints that are more vulnerable is triggering some deeper fear of the aging process that the patient wants to avoid. So he dampens down by eating more sugar or perhaps self-medicating with alcohol or marijuana, which of course causes the joint pain to worsen. For this we might consider a Yang Wei treatment:

- **SJ-5** on the left (postnatal male) opens the Yang Wei.

- The Yang Wei has a large trajectory with many points to choose from. You might consider the points that affect the joints like: **GB-29** (hips), **LI-14** (shoulders), **GB-21** (neck and shoulders).

- **GB-35** is the xi-cleft and that can be used to unblock the system and restore movement.

- **UB-63** is the first point on the channel and it is the xi-cleft point of the Urinary Bladder channel. This point unblocks Tai Yang and may provide some impulse towards movement.

- You might also look at **GB-20** or **GB-13**. GB-20 clears the sensory orifices and this may allow the patient to see his options more clearly. It will also treat the neck pain. GB-13 clears phlegmy thinking and calms the shen.

- You now need to decide if you want to add **GB-41**, the couple point, to this treatment. It can be used to provide the resources of Ming Men. It can also be used if the patient is having difficulty rotating at the waist or if the patient has low back pain too. You might want to consider the use of GB-41 to help the patient let go of the thoughts or emotions that are impeding movement into the future. In this way the added influence of the Dai Mai helps to release the old judgment he might have about himself. You choose the points on the trajectory that best reflect the specific pathology your patient is experiencing. You want to address both the physical and emotional symptoms in order to relieve the patient's suffering.

YANG QIAO

A 42-year-old male patient is suffering from lingering pain from an automobile accident last week. The neck pain is worse on the left and his upper back and hip are more painful on the right. His pain is aggravated by forward flexion and extension. This is not his first accident. He was in a very serious accident when he was younger, which should have made him more careful but he was in such a hurry to get to his next appointment and he was under the pressure of multiple deadlines. He drove too quickly and was too distracted to avoid the accident. This patient's musculoskeletal pain and his over-directed forward movement lead us to the Yang Qiao.

- **UB-62** on the right (side of most pain).

- **UB-59** xi-cleft point of the channel to unblock the circulation of qi and blood. This helps to relieve the pain but it also unblocks the impediments that keep us from being present in the moment.

- **GB-29** on the right for the hip pain. This engages shao yang and allows us to move with flexibility. It helps us to respond to external stimuli allowing us to change direction when necessary.

- **GB-20** on the left for the neck pain and also to help open the sensory orifices to see the world around us more clearly.

- You might also consider adding **ashi points** for pain and **Du-20** for increased awareness and back pain. You might also consider engaging the foot yang sinews by bleeding **UB-67** or stimulating the foot yang meeting point of the sinew channels **SI-18**.

YIN QIAO

Your 28-year-old female patient has been diagnosed with uterine fibroids. Her gynecologist says that they are small and she can wait to see if they change in size before deciding whether or not to have surgery to have them removed. She tells you that she really wants to look inward and figure out why she has developed these fibroids. She had a difficult childhood and she wants to let that go and take a stand for a future that is based more powerfully on who she is. She is taking some meditation classes but she is having difficulty sitting still. The accumulation in the abdomen and the desire to look inward might lead to you to the Yin Qiao.

- **Ki-6** the master point of the Yin Qiao can be done bilaterally to create stability and internal alignment or unilaterally to create circulation.

- **Ki-8** the xi-cleft point unblocks the system and helps to remove stagnation.

- **St-12** supports the descending of qi and fluids and will help the patient to slow down enough to look inward.

- **UB-1** can direct the vision inwards, strengthening the capacity for insight. If the patient is reluctant to allow you to needle UB-1 then UB-2 is an acceptable substitute. It is not as good as the UB-1 for insight, but it does direct energy towards the eyes especially if it is needled towards UB-1.

- Although it is not necessary you might consider adding a Ren point in the lower abdomen to help to resolve the fibroids and to regulate how the lower jiao distributes yin.

- If the childhood difficulties are related to the patient's relationship to their mother or primary caregiver then you might also add **Lu-7**, the couple point of the Yin Qiao and master point of the Ren Mai.

DAI MAI

A 40-year-old patient who is carrying some weight around the middle comes to you for chronic vaginal discharge. She has a history of sexual abuse. She is in therapy and she knows she needs some help releasing the old trauma so that she can move on with her life. She doesn't want the abuse to define her and stop her from having healthy relationships, with good boundaries.

This is a Dai Mai issue but in patients who have suffered violation of their boundaries I prefer to be gentle in how I release the Dai Mai. So it is likely that I would combine the Dai Mai with Ren Mai. Adding the Ren Mai creates a sense of safety and containment that allows for the Dai Mai to be drained in a kinder fashion.

- I might use the **Lu-7** with **GB-41** in the infinity loop. If the patient is more fragile or has fewer resources I might begin with the Ren and add the Dai Mai as the couple point. Otherwise I would use the GB-41 first and couple it with Lu-7.

- **Lv-13,** the influential point of the zang organs—this allows the yuan qi to be more easily disseminated by the zang organs, which in turn supports postnatal function, specifically the ability to transform and transport.

- Thread **GB-27** towards **GB-28**—this engages the storage function of the Dai Mai and allows for old hurts to be released.

- Thread **Ren-15** towards **Ren-14**, which calms the shen and opens the Bao Mai (uterine vessel), which is often damaged in cases of sexual abuse. Some patients with sexual abuse may not be comfortable with direct needling below the navel, so opening this loop between Ren-15 and Du-1 (Bao Mai) allows you to access the site of violation indirectly.

DAI MAI

Let's say you have a male patient with a history of anger management issues accompanied by chronic depression. This would be the type of depression that is recognized as anger turned inwards. He may be passive-aggressive in his relationships and prone to flare ups of heat due to frustration and emotional constraint that cause him to lose his temper.

- This patient would be robust enough that you can be more aggressive when using the Dai Mai, so you can easily begin with **GB-41** and use **SJ-5** on the opposite side. The contralateral use of these points will stimulate movement.

- **GB-37** is the luo point. This can be added if the patient is lacking in the courage to do what is needed in order to change or it might be used to help the patient see his options more clearly.

- **GB-29** might be used if the patient is rigid or lacking in flexibility or adaptability when required to change. These patients might dig their heels in and refuse to budge. GB-29 can initiate movement in the legs, helping the patient to step in a different direction.

- **GB-21** can be added to relax the energy moving into the arms, taking some of the fight out of the arms. I often use this point in angry patients who have clenched fists.

- **GB-20** might be used to clear the chaos (wind) from the head and help the patient to see things more clearly.

- **Du-24** calms the shen and opens the courtyard of spirit supporting the development of consciousness.

- If the patient is a phlegmy or obsessive thinker or if they are prone to rumination then you might also add **GB-13**. The Dai Mai has a very strong resonance with the Gall

Bladder channel and its coupled vessel, the Yang Wei also has a strong shao yang influence. The Yang Wei has many points that support the Dai Mai function and you can use any of them in a treatment like this. All you need is a good reason to add them and a clear understanding that any point you use should add to the intent instead of distracting from it.

Although these are all simulated cases I am sure many of you will have already seen patients who have some of these characteristics. The 8 EV give us a tool that can honor the curriculum, balance the emotions and relieve the symptoms that are causing the patient pain and suffering.

— CHAPTER 11 —

CASE STUDIES

When I teach, many of my students really appreciate having case studies to deepen their learning. It gives them a way to see the theory in action. In a classroom, I can create fictional cases that demonstrate the principles being taught just like I did in the previous chapter. I can use my imagination to create scenarios that will perfectly illustrate whatever it is I am teaching in that moment. In this chapter the cases are real. Identifying details have been altered to maintain the privacy of the patient and I have permission from all of those included to share their stories.

There is a problem in using real cases in a book. Real cases are about real people and real people are complex and nuanced and their suffering has sometimes taken many years to evolve into its current state. There is no way to include everything that may be significant to the diagnosis and understanding of the patient. Only the information that I considered essential at the time of treatment is included. This is the information that helped me to make a diagnosis and determine a treatment principle. So what the reader is really experiencing is my perspective and observations. The cases that follow are seen through my filters and the patients themselves may have a very different perspective on their experience. Some of these cases happened a long time ago and my perspective is different now and, one would hope, more refined.

I hope that including these cases will help you to understand my process in choosing and using these powerful vessels. The generous patients who gave their permission to use elements of their stories for the purpose of teaching each have their own stories to tell and I am well aware that what they read here might not resonate with their own experience of treatment. I hope they will forgive the liberties taken for the sake of education.

SANDRA: EARLY 60S, MARRIED, MEDICAL PROFESSIONAL

Sandra's chief complaint was low energy related to recovery from some type of stomach virus. This began several weeks before her first visit. In addition to the fatigue she was also experiencing muscle soreness. The muscle aches were previously related to side effects from the use of a medication. After stopping the medication the aching went away and then the aching returned with the stomach virus. The muscle pain was mild and it did not appear to interfere with Sandra's daily activities. Of greater concern was the fatigue, which the patient described as "a lack of reserve and feeling less resilient." The patient was also taking medication for low thyroid and medication for symptoms of menopause. In general, the patient has been active and healthy, a non-smoker and a social drinker. Even though the chief complaint was feeling a lack of reserves, the patient looks well put together and appears on the outside to have some vitality. The patient has also been taking medication for sleep. She reports that her tendency for overthinking keeps her from settling into sleep at night. The medication helps her to sleep but it does nothing to help the feeling of fatigue that has been plaguing her lately. The patient describes herself as not being very good at self-care. It is much easier for her to care for others. Sandra also mentioned that her digestion was weak and that seems to run in her family. She tries to eat well but is prone to indigestion and gas and bloating with some foods. Her tongue was pale-pink, dry with a few small horizontal cracks. The tip was narrow. Her pulse was weak, deep and thready throughout except the right middle position which was slightly soft and inflated.

Based on the given information I decided to treat the Ren Mai. Her digestive weakness, sleep difficulty and inability to embrace her self-care could all be addressed through the Ren Mai as well as the yin deficiency and fatigue.

On her first visit I needled Lu-7 and Ki-6 in an infinity loop; starting with Lu-7 on the left side, adding next Ki-6 on the right, then Ki-6 on the left and finishing with the right Lu-7. This in effect creates a figure 8 called an "infinity loop." Like the Mobius strip it is named after, this needling approach has a profoundly deep and archetypal effect that helps to regulate the polarity of yin and yang.

I added Ren-11 Jian Li/Strengthening the Interior to promote digestive function and to help with that feeling of being less resilient. Yes I could have used Ren-12 for the same purpose but upon palpation the Ren-11 had a distinct feeling of weakness, a lack of resilience.

I also needled St-36 to support the tonification of the Spleen, Stomach and qi and blood. The Stomach point I added was a he-sea point resonant with yuan qi. The Stomach channel itself has a very strong resonance with the Ren Mai based on the Stomach points on the face that are part of the Ren Mai pathway and also because the Ren Mai has a strong relationship with the Sea of Nutrition (St-30, St-36). The last point in the treatment was Du-24 Shen Ting/Spirit Courtyard. This point was added to support consciousness, calm the spirit and help sleep but also because it intersects with the stomach channel thereby strengthening the Ren Mai's relationship with digestive function by engaging the motive force of the Du Mai.

The idea was to get her to embrace her yin. My intent was to help her feel more nourished, to strengthen her digestion so she could produce more postnatal yin through the function of the stomach and then to use that yin to provide nourishment to her muscles to relieve the aching. I also hoped she would feel and enjoy the slower pace of yin.

On her second visit the patient reported feeling more like her "old self." Her pain was gone and her energy had returned. Her tongue had not changed but her pulse was less deep. So I repeated the Ren Mai treatment with some small modifications. I used Lu-7 and Ki-6 (infinity loop) with St-36. I then added Ren-6 to help circulate the qi in the middle and support the function of digestion. I also replaced Ren-11 with Ren-12 with the intent of creating more stability in the middle. I also added Ren-24 to stimulate salivation for digestion to begin in the mouth. I used Du-24 for the same reason as last time. The patient's energy continued to improve and her overall sense of well-being increased.

Several weeks later the patient over-exerted herself and had a flare up of an old injury. She was experiencing back pain, neck pain and right hip pain. She was also experiencing a headache that was worse on the right side. Her pulse was diaphragmatic (forceful between the first and second position) and her tongue was red at the tip. So even though I knew her history around self-care (Ren Mai) I decided it would be more helpful in this particular treatment to address the structure and her means for locomotion. She was over-extended into the world, trying to do too much.

For this condition, I used the Yang Qiao to address the musculoskeletal pain, qi and blood stagnation with heat. The Yang Qiao will also address the fact that the patient is over-extended into the world and not creating enough time for rest. You could say she is pushing too hard and that has caused the exterior to tighten up or brace. It also became clear to me that all the work we had done so far on the Ren Mai had increased her awareness of self. It was a step in the right direction that she decided to come for treatment when these old injuries began to surface into her awareness.

I began the treatment with UB-62 and UB-59 on the right side because most of her pain was on the right. UB-62 is the master point of the Yang Qiao and UB-59 is the xi-cleft point. In this way we created an opening for her circulation to be restored. Additional points included GB-29 on the right for the hip pain, UB-40 bilaterally and Hua Tuo Jia Ji points at the level of the sacrum up to the third lumbar vertebrae on the right—all for the back pain. Du-9 and UB-43 were added to open the diaphragm and release emotional constraint that was evident in her diaphragm pulse. I used GB-20 on the left to treat the headache and neck pain. Using it on the left helps balance the polarity from right to left. Sometimes when a patient has a headache at the time of treatment I will avoid using GB-20 on the affected side because I have seen it make a headache worse. In that case I might use GB-12 or GB-21. The last point used was Du-20 to engage the primal yang and calm the spirit.

The following week the patient was feeling much better. Her pain was gone leaving only a little stiffness in the neck and upper back but she seemed to be falling into the caregiver role again. She was worried that the pain was going to return when she had to travel to take care of a family member. She also reported that her digestion was sluggish again and she was experiencing some indigestion. Her tongue was still red at the tip. Working at the level of yuan qi is a process that unfolds over time. So often it is three steps forward, one step back.

I wanted to return to the Ren Mai since I felt that the underlying issue was a result of a weakness in resources provided by the Ren Mai. I was concerned that if I did not also address the musculoskeletal system the pathology would flare again, especially with the travelling and the physical over-exertion required to care for someone else. I combined the two vessels by making the figure 8/ infinity loop with Lu-7, Ki-6, UB-62 and completing the loop with SI-3—Lu-7 on the left, Ki-6 on the right, UB-62 on the left and SI-3 on the right.

I added to that treatment, St-36, Ren-6 for the digestive problems, Ren-13 for the indigestion and Du-24, Du-20 to calm the shen. This is a way of trying to create balance between yin and yang. It is also quite helpful in balancing the autonomic nervous system. It is a way to activate the microcosmic orbit (cycling energy between the Ren and Du Mai). It was my intent that she would not abandon herself completely in order to care for someone else.

She managed the trip quite well, only having some small discomfort that she was easily able to address and overcome. I still see the Ren Mai imbalance as the root problem, but I also anticipate that the closer we get to restoring balance in the Ren Mai the more we will have to work through a lifetime of compensation in the physical structure that pushes her to over-extend into the world. Sandra continues to see me intermittently when she feels the need.

I have, in the sharing of Sandra's story, focused on the psychological aspects of her suffering. The Ren Mai brings to the patient the capacity for self-care and self-love. That does not mean that I did not find her physiological symptoms important. My choice of the Ren Mai covered most of the physiological complaints the patient was experiencing on the first visit. Her primary physiological signs and symptoms were related to qi and yin deficiency and qi stagnation, all of which could be treated effectively using the Ren Mai. This is just another example of how the body and mind are not separate. The physiological symptoms reflect the deeper imbalances of the spirit.

Summary of treatments with points listed in the order they were inserted

- **Ren Mai**: Lu-7, Ki-6, Ren-11, St-36, Du-24.

- **Ren Mai**: Lu-7, Ki-6, Ren-6, Ren-12, Ren-24.

- **Yang Qiao**: UB-62, UB-59, UB-40, GB-29, Hua Tuo Jia Ji, Du-9, UB-43, GB-20, Du-20.

- **Ren + Yang Qiao**: Lu-7, Ki-6, UB-62, SI-3, St-36, Ren-6, Ren-13, Du-24, Du-20.

Remember, in the larger prescriptions many of the points were done only on one side to limit the number of needles and to stimulate circulation.

CATHERINE: 50S, FITNESS COACH

Catherine's chief complaint was a testament to her self-awareness. She came for treatment because she "felt stuck and needed to open up." Although she had some minor physical symptoms including some minor joint and muscle pain aggravated by exercise and intermittent digestive discomfort, she was clear that she wanted to focus on the emotional aspect of her health. Catherine felt that her "stuckness" began early in her life when she was unable to express the feelings of hurt, abandonment and disappointment in her relationship with her father. Her heart was broken early and she continued later in life to attract men who would also fail her. She had done much of the emotional work associated with this old hurt and she felt that she was ready to let go of the lingering energy that was keeping her from moving forward in her life and preventing her from attracting a healthy and fulfilling relationship. Catherine's body reflects that holding on. She has that "apple" shape that results from accumulation and holding in the trunk. Her arms and legs are much thinner in comparison to her trunk. On her first visit, her tongue was dusky (slightly darker) and the tip was a little red. Her tongue was also dry and narrow at the tip. This let me know that the emotional constraint she was experiencing was generating heat and depleting some of her fluid resources (yin). Her pulse was weaker in both kidney positions and the main force of the pulse was between the first and second positions (diaphragm). I determined that the Ren Mai would help her to direct her qi and support her ability to make deep and meaningful connections with herself and others. If she could feel worthy of self-love then attracting a loving relationship would come more easily. If she had been having anxiety about her experience or if she had unrealistic expectations, I might have chosen the Yin Wei first, because of the heartbreak. But since she had already done a lot of therapy, she had good awareness of her pattern. So by using the Ren Mai, I am, if you will, returning to the scene of the crime. I am going back to that time when the injury first occurred and I am trying to help her unlock the imprint caused by the early trauma.

I wanted to address the trauma caused by her father's perceived abandonment in childhood. To do that I decided to access the emotions and body memories in that first cycle of jing and release them so that she would no longer need to carry that burden. This can be done using the relationship that the Seven Po (Corporeal Souls) have to the seven/eight year cycles. The Seven Po reflect the seven stages of life and ideally as we move from one stage or cycle to another we "release" the old Po when the new Po arrives for the next stage of development. Any trauma in a particular stage may result in arrested development. This can cause a person's curriculum to become stuck or fixated at the stage when the trauma occurred. In Catherine's case that meant her ability to bond in relationship was traumatized by her father's abandonment in her first cycle of jing. To access those seven stages we can use either of the two vessels, the Ren and Du Mai, that most strongly govern the seven/eight year cycles of jing. Each of these vessels has a luo-collateral system that can hold trauma and emotions in latency until we have the resources, in later cycles, to address them. These luo vessels can be used to release old emotions and body memories from specific cycles that may be draining or obstructing vital resources. To release the trauma one uses the luo of either the Ren or Du and the specific point on the channel that is related to the cycle of jing one wants to open. Note that in both the Ren and Du, there is a break in the sequence. Du-4 is not needled out of respect for an individual's Destiny as it is disseminated through Ming Men and Ren-14 (Front-mu of the heart) is also not needled to show respect for the sovereignty of the heart.

Po treatment	Ren Mai	Du Mai
Access to the seven/ eight year cycles	**Ren-15** (luo point)	Du-1 (luo point)
First cycle of jing	**Ren-13**	Du-2
Second cycle	Ren-12	**Du-3**
Third cycle	Ren-11	**Du-5**
Fourth cycle	Ren-10	Du-6
Fifth cycle	Ren-9	Du-7
Sixth cycle	Ren-7	Du-8
Seventh cycle	Ren-6	Du-9

Catherine's first treatment was as follows: Ren-15 (luo point), Ren-13 (represents the first cycle), Lu-7 and Ki-6 in a figure 8 (infinity loop) and Ren-24. The Ren-24 was added to help her receive the nourishment of love that was her birthright.

After this treatment, the patient experienced movement in her physical body and her emotional process. She found her emotions to be more accessible and even went to a sibling to talk about their experiences in childhood.

Between the first and second treatment, Catherine went to a retreat in the mountains where a fire and the resulting smoke caused her to develop some sinus problems and vertigo. I did not want to stray too far from the Ren Mai as I felt it was the key to her emotional constraint but I did not want to ignore the obstruction of the yang channels from the exposure to the smoke.

In the second treatment I added the Du Mai to the treatment to address the obstruction of the yang channels of the head. The treatment began with: (L) Lu-7, (R) Ki-6, (L) UB-62 and (R) SI-3 done in the figure 8.

I added to that: Du-24 (three needles, like an arrow pointed posteriorly towards Du-20) to open the sinuses, St-7 (to descend the energy from the head), Ren-12, Ren-6 and St-40. The stomach channel has a strong affinity for the Ren Mai that can be seen in the channel pathway around the mouth and also by its association with the Sea of Nutrition.

After this treatment the vertigo went away and the patient felt calmer and more grounded. She became more acutely aware of her belly and the extra weight she was carrying around the waist. She recognized that this weight was a form of protection but she felt she was ready to let it go, even if it meant being more aware of her feelings.

Following the patient's lead, this treatment continued to support the Ren Mai but I added the Dai Mai to support the awareness around the middle. I began the treatment with Lu-7 on the left and GB-41 on the right. Ren-11 (Jian Li/Strengthen the Interior) was used to support the function of the middle jiao and Ren-6 to circulate and support qi function. To engage the energy of the prenatal Dai Mai, I used: St-25 and Sp-15 both found at the level of the umbilicus and therefore on the pathway of the prenatal Dai Mai. Sp-9 was added to gently drain the dampness obstructing the functioning of the middle jiao. Of course, this treatment does not make you lose 20 pounds of abdominal fat overnight but it is a way to bring consciousness to the reasons that the weight lingers and may be resistant to diet and exercise.

Catherine continued to see me once or twice a month as she worked through the process of letting go of the past. She seems happier and less stuck in her history. She returns for treatment when she is aware of resistance. In this way, she determines how quickly her jing unfolds.

Summary of treatments

- **Po treatment**: Ren-15, Ren-13 + Lu-7, Ki-6, Ren-24.

- **Ren + Du**: Lu-7, Ki-6, UB-62, SI-3, Du-24, St-7, Ren-12, Ren-6, St-40.

- **Ren + Dai**: Lu-7, GB-41, Ren-11, Ren-6, St-25, Sp-15, Sp-9.

JAMES: LATE 40S, CREATIVE PROFESSIONAL

James came to see me with acute low back pain brought on he said by bending over to pick something up. His pain was centralized on the spine and he described it as feeling gripping and very unstable. Normally I would treat this kind of injury with the primary channels restoring qi and blood flow and reducing local spasm. James told me two things that made me decide to use the 8 EV. The first thing he told me was that he had a history of low back pain. This was a recurring pattern for him. The second thing he told me was that prior to injuring his low back his stress levels were through the roof. Not only was he extremely busy at work, having to put in long hours under a lot of pressure but he was also going through a difficult divorce. He was very sensitive to palpation and was having an elevated response to external stimuli. He was basically a little twitchy like he was waiting for the rug to be pulled out from under him. Although the back pain was not as bad as when he first bent down, he was having difficulty sitting down and he could not take off his socks without debilitating pain. Upon palpation his mid and upper back were very tight and he complained that his right hand tingled when he picked up his cell phone. So his whole back and neck were affected by this injury and complicated by the level of stress. He was being overwhelmed by his current circumstances. What he really needed was a vacation from his life but that wasn't going to happen anytime soon. I decided to use the Yang Qiao to create better circulation in his musculoskeletal system and at the same time help his body to deal with the fact the he was over-extended and, basically, that he was living a life that was not unlike a runaway freight train. He was so over-extended that he could not feel the warnings that his back had been giving to him before it went on strike. The bending over that resulted in severe pain was the last straw. The body had been giving him signals for a while that he had been steadfastly ignoring in order to fulfill his obligations. The requirements of his life would not allow him to move voluntarily into a yin state (vacation mode) but he needed to be able to find some balance in how much yang energy he was directing outwards. He also needed to be able to release some of the emotional constraint that was preventing the healthy circulation of qi and blood. I used the Yang Qiao to try to slow down the train and restore his circulation.

I used the master point UB-62 on the left and all of the other points were used bilaterally (except the Du Mai points of course) in order to create a sense of balance and stability that was currently missing in his life. UB-59 (xi-cleft) point was used to unblock the channel and restore the movement of qi and blood. UB-40, Yao Yan, Du-4 and Du-3 were used because of the back pain. Du-9 and UB-43 were added for the emotional constraint. Du-9 opens the diaphragm and regulates the liver and Gall Bladder. UB-43 is the outer shu of the pericardium, which can release emotional constraint and is frequently used for chronic recurring conditions. Du-16 and Du-20 were used to help regulate his nervous system and calm the shen.

A week later I saw him for a second treatment and he was much improved. His pain was significantly less but he was still a little twitchy. So I did the same treatment with a small modification. I did not use UB-43 and Du-16 but I added GB-20 to open his sensory orifices and relax his neck and upper back. Because GB-20 expels wind it can help when patients are challenged by the chaos or unpredictability of change.

He scheduled another appointment but later cancelled it because he was feeling so much better. I am certain that is in part because his work schedule makes it difficult for him to come for treatment but it is my hope that he will come for treatment before his back goes on strike again. He is aware that many of his current stressors will not last forever. I hope that he will be able to avoid the severity of pain and dysfunction by catching it sooner next time. Ultimately, he knows he needs to slow down and deal with the stress. Perhaps he will be able to do that soon but in the meantime he is able to return to work and fulfill his obligations, which is what he wanted from his treatments.

Summary of treatments

- **Yang Qiao**: UB-62, UB-59, UB-40, Yao Yan, Du-3, Du-4, Du-9, UB-43, Du-16, Du-20.

- **Yang Qiao**: Remove UB-43 and Du-16, add GB-20 (for the winds of change).

ANN: LATE 30S, CREATIVE PROFESSIONAL

Ann's chief complaint was numbness and tingling in the arms, legs and face. She said that this was associated with an auto-immune type of anemia that she had been diagnosed with a couple of years ago. She had been getting some improvement in her symptoms by having monthly vitamin B12 shots. Additional symptoms included dry mouth, chest pain, palpitations, restless sleep with nightmares, depression, stomach problems, nausea, diarrhea, thirst, worry, being easy to anger and being easily startled. Her libido was decreased and her memory was poor. Her pulse was very thready and her tongue was slightly pale-dusky and the edges were slightly red. She seemed anxious during the interview and she was fidgety. I felt when watching her that if she could relax and breathe more deeply, the stillness would bring her to a place where her circulation would be freer. In Ann we see what happens to our circulation when our yin resources are depleted. When we lose the ballast of yin and blood the body will often lock down to create stability. This is often related to the function of the pericardium. When we are blood deficient, the pericardium is forced to be more diligent in its protection. It is like how bodyguards react when the person they are guarding is shot. They are always vigilant and prepared but when their person is wounded or weakened they go into overdrive. Everything and everyone becomes a threat. In Ann's case she was not aware of how much tension she had in her neck and upper back. She was also not aware of how little she was breathing.

This is another patient who might have been served by the Yin Wei or the Ren Mai, as they both treat blood deficiency. So, I had to choose between the two. At the time this came down to instinct or perhaps experience. There was something about her demeanor that made me think more of the Ren Mai than the Yin Wei. There was a subtle collapse in the chest as her shoulders were rolled slightly forward that is more resonant with the Ren Mai. She lacked tension along the diaphragm and there was something about the way she spoke about the numbness that was a little disconnected. So, I decided to start with the Ren Mai, knowing that I could move on to the Yin Wei if I didn't get the results.

Her first treatment began with: Lu-7 and Ki-6 in a figure 8. Ki-8 was added as the xi-cleft point of the Yin Qiao. This point can unblock the abdomen and help people to trust their guts. To this I added Ren-6 and Ren-13 to regulate the digestive qi and Du-24 to calm the spirit and open the consciousness. Ren-13 is also very useful in calming anxiety and supporting deeper respiration.

Her numbness improved, as did her mood, so we continued with the Ren Mai. On her third treatment her pulse changed. She had been doing a lot of physical work under a deadline and was suffering from pain and stiffness in the neck and upper back, which was worse on the right and her hips were aching. Her treatment was changed to address the physical discomfort of over-exertion: (R) UB-62 plus bilateral UB-59 (xi-cleft), GB-29, SI-10, GB-20 and Du-24. This treatment eased the physical pain.

In the following months Ann would come for treatment every three to four weeks and we returned for the most part to the Ren Mai. Over the course of six months not only did the numbness improve and rarely recurred but also her body awareness, confidence and clarity in her work all increased. Once she had a deeper connection to herself and an ability to better trust that connection, she was able to feel more comfortable and relaxed in her body. Also, as the Sea of Yin the Ren Mai was able to support the blood, which was not nourishing the muscles resulting in the numbness and tingling.

Summary of treatments

- **Ren + Yin Qiao**: Lu-7, Ki-6, Ki-8, Ren-6, Ren-13, Du-24.
- **Yang Qiao**: UB-62, UB-59, GB-29, SI-10, GB-20, Du-24.

DANIEL: 60, SELF-EMPLOYED

Daniel first came to me with a severely compromised respiratory system. He had a cough, wheezing, shortness of breath with exertion and he was also losing his voice. The most recent episode of these symptoms began six months prior to his first visit with me but the problem originally began almost 20 years earlier and was severe enough to require hospitalization. He has been given no firm medical diagnosis although his doctor suspects he has asthma related to allergies. He has been given a variety of inhalers but so far the only thing that has given him any kind of relief is prednisone. The prednisone relieves most of his symptoms while he is taking it and for about four days afterwards.

With this very long history of respiratory issues that have been resistant to treatment I felt the need to find out more about his constitution and early childhood history. He suffered birth trauma when he was dropped on his head at the time the doctor was first handing him to his mother. Because of this trauma he was taken away and was therefore unable to bond to his mother. In addition to that trauma, his father passed away when he was 18 months old, which then made his mother understandably even more unavailable. Soon after, his grandparents took over his care. His breathing problems first started to show up at 13 years of age in the form of some post-nasal drip and mild wheezing. This began at the time that he was sent away to boarding school.

Daniel describes himself as liking control and order and notes that he is currently having difficulty completing a project because of a driving need for the project to be perfect before he turns it in.

His tongue was dusky-red with a narrow tip and his pulse was a Ren Mai pulse bilaterally. I wanted to help Daniel remove the imprint of the birth trauma and help him to create some closure on the insufficient bonding with his mother. To that end, I did a Po treatment using the first cycle of jing (Ren-15 and Ren-13). It was my intent that the body memory of those earlier traumas would be released and no longer have a hold on his ability to regulate his breathing. I added to that treatment Lu-7 and Ki-6 in the figure 8 (infinity loop) using the Ren Mai to help create closure on the earlier traumas and to help ease the need for control and perfection. St-36 was added to help transform some of the dampness. Lu-2 was threaded to Lu-1 to help Daniel receive and Du-24 to open his consciousness to the possibility that his history was affecting his ability to take the world in. After the first treatment he noticed that the cough was a little better and he was urinating more, especially at night.

After that treatment he remembered a time in his 30s when he felt so helpless while watching his then wife suffer the pain and fear of breast cancer. The cancer had spread to her lungs and was causing terrible fluid accumulation that was making it so difficult for her to breathe. She eventually passed away from the ravages of this disease and he was left in his grief.

After his first treatment his pulse and tongue remained the same. During this next treatment we focused on his inability to deal with the emotions surrounding his wife's suffering and his sense of helplessness. I decided to use the Yin Wei to see if I could support his respiration by opening his chest and easing his heart and pericardium. In effect, I wanted to help him heal his broken heart. I used Pc-6 on the left and Sp-4 on the right to open the Yin Wei and support the opening of his chest and the asthma with the Chong Mai. I added to that Sp-10 on the right to harmonize the blood and emotions and Ki-9 on the left to unblock the Yin Wei (xi-cleft point). To support movement in the chest I added Lv-14 and Lu-2 threaded to Lu-1. To support consciousness I used Du-24.

After this treatment he had improvement for about three days, then his symptoms returned pretty severely. He decided to start back on the prednisone and when he returned for his next visit about two weeks later, he had finished the prednisone for several days. He had plans at that time to do one more round of the prednisone because he felt the relief from the physical symptoms was allowing for the spiritual part of the work to emerge. He was acutely aware of the emotion arising from his father's birthday anniversary and the recent death by suicide of a young friend. Physiologically, he was more acutely aware of a stuck sensation in his epigastrium and a mid to upper back constraint or tension in the muscles of his chest that made him feel as though he wanted to "spread his wings." In an effort to help him to free up his back so he could "fly," I did a Yang Qiao treatment on him with moving cups on his upper back. This treatment helped for about a week and then he had a crisis. He almost went to the emergency room because he became acutely aware of a deep tightness and discomfort deep in the center of his chest (he pointed to the Kidney shu points). He said that was accompanied by a tightness "like a wrapper" around his chest to his mid-back. These symptoms are reflective of pathology in the Chong Mai and Yin Wei. Once the blood stasis was cleared from the exterior he was better able to feel the blood stasis in the interior.

His pulse was deep (Chong Mai) and his tongue had developed a turbid coat. I used the Chong Mai and the Yin Wei to treat the interior. I used Sp-4 on the left and Pc-6 on the right to open the Chong and support it with the Yin Wei. I added St-40 to open the chest and clear the turbidity reflected in his tongue coat and Ki-16 to bring the energy down into the legs. On his chest I used Ki-22 (zhi and water point) needled in towards the sternum to help consolidate and Ki-26 (Po and metal point) needled outward to support expansion in the chest and Ren-17 to influence the movement of qi in the chest. The last point added was Ren-23 to open the throat and support communication.

As of writing this chapter, I had seen him one more time and at that visit we continued with the Chong Mai treatment. He had some improvement in the chest pain. He states the cough was about the same but, objectively, I felt as though he was actually coughing significantly less than on previous visits and the nature of the cough was less deep. He said in the ten days between this treatment and the last he had several past life experiences that were helping him to understand that he had several lifetimes of dealing with his ability to engage the world on his own terms. He recognized that there was work to do and that the respiration problem was an opportunity to embrace those lessons. So we will continue to work on his respiration and the circulation in his chest. We will continue to work on his long history of heart ache and even the possibility that in previous lives his need to follow his heart caused him much suffering. His relationship to his inability to breathe was much more relaxed and less fraught with fear and doubt. We will likely continue to treat the Chong Mai as a way of dealing with the circulation in his chest but also as a way of helping him to rediscover who he is. The Chong Mai is also a way to negotiate those past life experiences and the early childhood trauma that has shaped his current struggles.

Summary of treatments

- **Po treatment**: Ren-15, Ren-13 + Lu-7, Ki-6, St-36, Lu-2 threaded towards Lu-1, Du-24.

- **Yin Wei**: Pc-6, Sp-4, Sp-10, Ki-9, Lv-14, Lu-2 threaded towards Lu-1, Du-24.

- **Yang Qiao**: Right UB-62, (L) GB-41, UB-23, UB-20, Du-9, UB-43, UB-13, Ding Chuan, Du-20.

- **Chong + Yin Wei**: Sp-4, Pc-6, St-40, Ki-16, Ki-22, Ki-26, Ren-17, Ren-23.

SUSAN: LATE 30S, HOMEMAKER AND SELF-EMPLOYED

Susan is a slender, well-groomed young woman who on her initial visit was bright, pleasant and friendly with the associates in the office. You might even say she was cheerful. However, even before seeing her chart for the first time or doing her intake, I couldn't help noticing how skittish she was. Her movements were quick and she seemed a little more vigilant than was necessary for safety's sake. Her eyes were full of light but very wide and outwardly directed, as if she was trying to fully capture the room and its inhabitants. Those observations made perfect sense when I saw her intake form and the chief complaint was anxiety. Her response to the question asking her when this complaint began was: "unknown." She was experiencing palpitations and sleep problems including nightmares and this difficulty sleeping had caused her to feel tired easily. She was currently taking Xanax as needed for the anxiety, a selective serotonin reuptake inhibitor (SSRI) for depression and Chinese herbs given to her by another practitioner. Her tongue was pale and a little dusky (darker) around the edges and the coat was thin and white. Her pulse was mostly weak and a little bit thinner than you might expect with her thin build.

We began with a Po treatment for the first cycle of jing. I used Ren-15 and Ren-13 for trauma in the first cycle of jing. This was supported by Lu-7 and Ki-6 done bilaterally with a figure 8 starting with Lu-7 on the left. Because of her skittishness I added only two additional points: Ki-2 for fear and anxiety to move the energy away from the sensory orifices and into the feet for grounding. This was done on the right side only to limit the number of needles. On the left I did UB-2 for the outwardly directed eyes (UB-2). UB-1 might have been preferable from a function point of view but I felt that it would have caused more anxiety.

The patient did very well after the treatment. She was very tired immediately after the treatment but she did sleep better for the next few days. She reported still being very sensitive to the environment and since the treatment she was more acutely aware of the energy focused around her eyes. She then said she would like to be able to "see a future without anxiety." Her menses was only two days in length with light bleeding. I continued with the Ren Mai hoping to give her a sense of yin-stillness and knowing that the lack of yin vital substance (blood) forced her awareness to be unanchored and outwardly directed. I used Lu-7 on the left and Ki-6 on the right with Ki-2, Lv-8, UB-2, all done bilaterally and Du-24 to calm the shen and relax the tension around her sensory orifices.

By her third treatment her anxiety was down to 2/10 and she was sleeping better and feeling more grounded. She managed her anxiety very well until life got more stressful and then it would resurface. At one point the anxiety flared up and the patient reported she felt "manic." She said she was worried about a trip she would be taking with her children that weekend that would require her to drive on the freeway. Her anxiety was really bad if she had to do any freeway driving. For this treatment I used the Lu-7 and Ki-6 in the figure 8 to create some containment and balance. I added to that Ki-8 on the right. Ki-8 is the xi-cleft point of the Yin Qiao and as such unblocks the Yin Qiao and helps patients to trust themselves. Its name Jiaoxin is sometimes translated as Exchange of Trust. Ki-4 was used on the left. As the luo point of the kidney channel it helps to relieve the fear that is triggered when one fears for their life or the lives of loved ones. I added stomach points to deal with the manic feelings, remembering that the stomach channel has a strong resonance with the function of the Ren Mai. The particular stomach points I used were St-36 and St-25. St-36 supports the transforming function of the middle jiao and stabilizes the middle and St-25 the front mu of the Large Intestine helps patients to let go. Its position on the abdomen at the level of the navel means that St-25 also contributes to stability. After this treatment Susan was able to make the drive with her children on the freeway without any panic or anything other than mild anxiety. I continue to treat Susan off and on as other health conditions arise but she is much more relaxed and less prone to feelings of anxiety. She has learned over time how to take care of herself in a way that supports her emotional health. She still struggles with a tendency towards anxiety but is less easily overwhelmed. We have been working a lot on diet lately, especially as it relates to her insulin resistance and a tendency towards systemic inflammation. As is often true with patients who have blood deficiency and emotional distress, the underlying weakness in the spleen and stomach is a contributing factor.

Summary of treatments

- **Po treatment**: Ren-15, Ren-13 + Lu-7, Ki-6, Ki-2, UB-2.

- **Ren Mai**: Lu-7, Ki-6, Ki-2, Lv-8, UB-2, Du-24.

- **Ren Mai**: Lu-7, Ki-6, Ki-8, Ki-4, St-36, St-25.

MARCIA: EARLY 40S, CREATIVE PROFESSIONAL

I first saw Marcia over 15 years ago. I had not been focusing my practice on the 8 EV at the time. When Marcia first saw me she did not have a chief complaint. She was a fit and healthy young woman who had some small complaints but mostly she was interested in dealing with health maintenance and reducing the effects of stress. Her early treatments were typical TCM treatments using the primary channel system. She came irregularly, mostly when she had time between projects and she was pleased with the results. For someone who actually hated the insertion of the needles, she loved the effects. Eventually a few years in, I began to see a pattern emerge. She had gone a while between projects and she was beginning to be stressed about money. As a person who pursued spiritual development she knew that this worry was a waste of her energy. She also knew she would be able to make enough money to pay her bills. She was also aware that the lack of work may be an indicator of her need to examine whether or not the work she was currently engaged in was the best way to fully express who she was. So we decided to approach this awareness through the 8 EV.

From a physical point of view, Marcia was suffering from a chronic pain in her wrists and forearms and a little pain off and on in her shoulders. She attributed this to her yoga practice. She also had some fatigue that was worse after eating. So there was definitely a Yang Ming component to the stagnation.

I felt that the money fears were first circuit issues related to the Lung, Large Intestine, Stomach and Spleen, which represent the struggles that we have with survival and the fact that at birth we are defenseless and dependent on those around us for our survival needs. This stage of development is where we have fear associated with deprivation. This is about not having enough— enough food, shelter, protection...and ultimately love. It is the stage early in life where we have to figure out what we have to do to get what we want or need.

This translates for me into the Ren Mai. Since the Ren Mai is the vessel that gifts us with yin resources, when we feel a lack of those resources we are feeling a primal fear. This theory was supported by the wrist and arm pain as the Ren Mai has a very strong connection to Yang Ming through the stomach channel. It was also resonant with Marcia's fatigue that was worse after eating, since the Ren Mai has a connection to the Sea of Nutrition (Sea of Ying).

So her first 8 EV treatment was: Lu-7 and Ki-6 in the figure 8 to open the Ren Mai and create a sense of stability in the middle. Added to that was St-36, Zu San Li/Leg 3 Miles, which supports the generation of postnatal resources in a way that means we can be assured that we can keep walking. On the abdomen I used the Four Doors: St-25 with Ren-12 and Ren-6. For this treatment, these points do three things: they create stability in the middle, they strengthen the capacity for transformation and through this transformation they support the generation of resources (qi and blood). For the arm pain, I added LI-10, which of course is a local point, but in addition to that its name Shou San Li/Arm 3 Miles means that it can be used effectively with St-36 for generalized tonification. Finally Du-24 was added to calm the shen and open consciousness.

By now many of you will be wondering why I keep using Du-24 to calm the shen rather than the more commonly used Yintang. My students will now recognize this as a "soap box" moment. Here I go, stepping up on my soap box to say, in my humble opinion, I find Yintang to be both overused and sometimes even ill-advised if your goal is developing consciousness and increased awareness. I have noticed with some of the patients who have had acupuncture prior to seeing me, a distinct awareness of the flood of neurotransmitters that are released with that point. Yes, it is calming but it is also for many addictive. I have had patients lying on the table actually tapping the point on their foreheads and saying things like: "Are you going to use this point? I really like this point. It really makes me relax. I think it makes my treatment work better." Not unlike a junkie saying if I could just have a hit, I'll be able to deal with everything better.

I think Yintang is a very powerful point and I do use it but only when I feel that it is the most appropriate point for the patient. I do not like to use it to knock my patient out or flood their system with happy chemicals. I appreciate the acu-stone that often comes with a good treatment as well as the next guy, but I would rather have the gift of increased self-awareness. Some people when they come for treatment are just looking for a mini vacation. This is a good reason to use Yintang. I also use it to stimulate the pituitary or support the opening of the third eye. But in the patients I work with who want to have a deeper awareness and an opportunity to learn and grow from their treatments, I usually avoid it. Okay, getting off the soap box now.

Back to Marcia's treatment. After this Ren Mai treatment, her wrist and arm pain was greatly relieved for a while (several days) and although the fear associated with not working as much was still present, she felt as though she was less reactive to the fear. I began to alternate the Ren Mai treatments with luo-collateral treatments for the first circuit. Those first circuit treatments were Lu-7 on the right, Li-6 on the left, St-40 on the left and Sp-4 on the right. These were not 8 EV treatments but rather a way to use the luo-collaterals to support the function of the 8 EV by helping the patient to "vent" or let go of the emotional process stuck at this early level of development. This combination of treatments proved to be very effective for Marcia. Not only was she able to let go of her fear of not having enough but also her energy opened up and she started attracting work again.

I see Marcia periodically. She is currently working very hard so she has to carve out time for her treatments. She is still working towards finding work that helps her to pay her bills but also feeds her soul.

Summary of treatments

- **Ren Mai**: Lu-7, Ki-6, St-36, St-25, Ren-12, Ren-6, LI-10, Du-24.

- **First circuit Po treatment**: Lu-7, LI-6, St-40, Sp-4.

JANET: EARLY 40S, SALES

Janet's chief complaint was insomnia. This was an ongoing problem for Janet for which she had been prescribed Sonata. The current episode had started six days previous to her initial visit. She described her sleep as insufficient (only a few hours) and restless. In addition to the sleep problems she also struggled with depression for which she had been prescribed Prozac (Fluoxetine) and Abilify (Aripiprazole). She had recently stopped taking the Abilify due to severe side effects. She also had the following symptoms: sinus problems, indigestion, heartburn, excessive appetite, sugar cravings and night sweats. I expected her tongue to have redness but it was pale overall with a greasy coat that was somewhere between white and yellow. Her pulse was weak and deep.

Based on the additional digestive and sinus issues and her pulse, I decided to use the Chong Mai and the Yin Wei together to treat the sleep and the depression. I was hoping that supporting the postnatal qi would help restore the relationship between the heart and kidneys. I used Sp-4 with contralateral Pc-6 to which I added St-40 to open the chest and reduce the phlegm, Sp-10 to harmonize the blood, Sp-15 to support the digestive function (Yin Wei), Ki-25 (front shu of heart, Chong Mai) and Du-24 to calm the shen and ease the depression.

This treatment did not help Janet sleep. She saw her MD and he gave her Xanax and she said it helped. She did not want to take it long term. She said that since her treatment she had become aware of overwhelming sadness. She had felt that since stopping the Abilify, but she was feeling it more deeply. She found the increased feelings stressful, which may have had an impact on her sleep. I changed her treatment to the Ren Mai in the hopes of calming and nourishing and supporting her ability to deal with her emotions.

This treatment included Lu-7 and Ki-6 in the figure 8, Du-24, Lu-2 threaded to Lu-1 to help deal with the sadness, Ren-17 and Sp-8 (Da Ji/Earth Mechanism) to support the Spleen's ability to process both food and emotions.

Shortly after this treatment (a few days) the patient developed an upper respiratory tract infection for which she took antibiotics. Once the infection resolved, the feelings of sadness were gone.

From this point onward my focus was on the depression and the uncomfortable feelings in the chest and abdomen that the patient associated with emotional distress. Even though she felt as though she was experiencing these emotions, she presented with a flat affect. Her experiences seemed to be much internalized and not outwardly expressed. I worked to create balance in the Ren and Du in the hopes of giving her sufficient yang to express her internal struggle.

I used: Lu-7, Ki-6, UB-62 and SI-3 in a figure 8 with Ren-15, Ren-4, Du-24 and Du-20. These treatments continued with small variations for several months. I continued to use the Lu-7, Ki-6, UB-62 and SI-3 and also two points on the Ren Mai and two points on the Du Mai. The points on the trajectory of the Ren and Du would change according to the patient's current symptoms. The patient's affect was significantly improved and her sleep was also better. In general, she seemed happier and her mood was more stable. During these later treatments I really began to enjoy the patient's sense of humor which was more apparent than when we first met.

Summary of treatments

-   **Chong + Yin Wei**: Sp-4, Pc-6, St-40, Sp-10, Sp-15, Ki-25, Du-24.

-   **Ren Mai**: Lu-7, Ki-6, Du-24, Lu-2 threaded to Lu-1, Ren-17, Sp-8.

-   **Ren + Du**: Lu-7, Ki-6, UB-62, SI-3 + Ren-15, Ren-4, Du-24, Du-20.

DAVID: MIDDLE AGE, WRITER

David's chief complaint was anxiety. This anxiety had lingered for the last six months and began several years after the death of his spouse. David was on the thin side and his demeanor was quiet and gentle. His tongue was pale, small and had teeth marks. His pulse was a Ren Mai pulse. He also complained of sinus congestion with weather changes, stomach problems, particularly nausea-related anxiety, headache, dizziness and frequent urination, especially at night. He was prescribed Lorazepam for the anxiety and found it helpful but did not want to be dependent on it to function.

In his relationship he had spent the last 22 years as his spouse's caretaker. Even with the stress of caretaking, he had no previous history of anxiety, his sleep was good and he had no awareness of any childhood trauma.

Due to his history as a caretaker and the confirming pulse, I decided to use the Ren Mai. His first treatment included Lu-7 and Ki-6 in a figure 8, Ren-12, Ren-14 and Du-24.

His second visit was two weeks later and by then he had reduced his medication by 50 percent. He was glad he was able to do this but it did result in a slight increase in anxiety. We continued to treat the Ren Mai with some small modifications.

Two months later the anxiety was much less in general and now seemed to be triggered by social events. He also experienced the anxiety lower in the belly now and sometimes in social settings he would get a little dizzy or light-headed. His pulse was thin and deeper and his tongue was pale with teeth marks. I decided to switch from the Ren Mai to the Chong Mai using Sp-4 with contralateral Pc-6, adding points to support the stomach function and points to help with the dizziness. Three months later he discontinued treatment because he was feeling much better. He was still decreasing his medication and had very few episodes of anxiety.

Summary of treatments

- **Ren Mai**: Lu-7, Ki-6, Ren-12, Ren-14, Du-24.

- **Chong Mai**: Sp-4, Pc-6, St-40, Sp-10, Ki-16, Ki-23, Du-24, Du-20.

- **Chong Mai**: Sp-4, Pc-6, Sp-10, Ki-16, GB-20, Du-24, Du-20.

A word about the treatments. You may have noticed a preponderance of Ren Mai treatments in the cases above. That definitely reflects my practice. It is not that the other vessels are less useful or that pathology in those vessels is rare. After practicing and teaching for nearly 20 years, one of the truths I have noticed is that most acupuncturists attract certain types of patients. I am sure there are many reasons for that. I know that these days my patient base is much different than it was 15 years ago. So, in part that may have something to do with building knowledge and capacity. Most of my patients have conditions that are much more complex than they used to be. I rarely get new patients who have things like tennis elbow or whiplash from a car accident. Even my acute back pain patients have some significant emotional distress or evolutionary pressure associated with their pain.

In part, it may also be about how you get referrals. These days most of my new patients come referred from other acupuncturists or psychotherapists. That was not true 15+ years ago. These patients are much more likely to have pathology in the first ancestry. They typically have not responded well to other treatment and they often have a history of trauma. That history lends itself to treatment of the Chong, Du or Ren.

For many of you it may also be about how you market your practice or how you specialize. I often say my specialty chose me. I did not set out to become the type of practitioner that I am. I did not necessarily want to specialize, as many believe, in the treatment of psycho-emotional disorders. I prefer to think of my practice as one that is firmly rooted in the effect of existential crises on health and well-being but how would one even begin to explain that to potential patients? So these days, when people ask I say that I treat stress-induced illness. Most people have some understanding that stress has a profound impact on health. The 8 EV are powerful tools for this.

There is another reason for the preponderance of Ren Mai treatments in my practice. These prenatal vessels are about how jing unfolds and this is an archetypal process. Each of these vessels has an archetypal resonance that supports the unfolding. If the patient is able to embrace the archetype and learn the lesson the archetype brings then they are able to move through it. If they are not able to embrace it then they will continue to be stuck and their suffering will linger.

As practitioners we have knowledge and skill to diagnose and treat illness but we are also responsible for creating a therapeutic environment in which the possibility for change exists. When we do this, we do this from who we are. Some people embrace the archetype of the healer by wearing a white coat and stethoscope. This symbolic image evokes a sense of trust and confidence in some patients. It helps them to feel as though they are in good and capable hands. Others might be uncomfortable with the symbol of the "white coat." They may feel it projects an air of authority and what they are looking for is someone who is willing to work with them in a partnership that is more equal and less authoritarian. Perhaps in their past they were misunderstood or mistreated by someone in a white coat.

Some practitioners embrace the archetype of the Du Mai when they practice. These practitioners either consciously or unconsciously embrace the archetype of the Father. They are able to provide a structure that helps tell patients what they must do to restore their health. Through that archetype they are able to instill confidence in the patient that helps them to feel courageous in the active pursuit of their health.

I, for a long list of reasons, embrace or perhaps it is more accurate to say embody the archetype of the Ren Mai. This at first began unconsciously for me and in the beginning it was uncomfortable and frustrating. I am a Mother to a wonderful young man and that is a large part of my identity but I had no desire to be Mother to many. I really don't consider myself to be "motherly." So I resisted the archetype. I have three younger brothers and I used to jokingly say that I was my father's oldest son. I felt much more secure in the realm of logic and action, and when I was younger I was well-appreciated for my intellect. So this was a safe and comfortable place to work from. Unfortunately, early in my practice, I attracted people who did not respond well to this "fatherly" archetype embodied in a female body. I learned how to embrace the "motherly" side of myself to create an environment that was most therapeutic for these patients.

These days, I resist less. I have come to a place where I understand that the reason that archetype is so effective for me is that I am driven to see my patients as unbroken. When I look at them, I look through the eyes of a mom. I try to focus on their unique perfection, not the pathology that is causing the suffering. I believe that this helps my patients to feel their worthiness through the eyes of the Mother. I believe it helps to remind them that they, like everyone else, are deserving of unconditional love. So because I have embraced this archetype, I attract patients who can benefit from this archetype. Thus, I do a lot of Ren Mai treatments.

When you begin to use these archetypal vessels you may consciously or unconsciously embrace the nature of a particular vessel. This means that you may see your patients through the lens of a particular vessel. I have a friend who does a lot of Chong Mai treatments. He has a sort of spiritual or shamanic energy to him that is uniquely suited for these treatments.

So if you decide to use these vessels in your treatments, they will offer you the same opportunity for your jing to unfold as you are offering your patients. They will, if you let them, change you. They will give you an avenue for becoming more of who you are.

—— CHAPTER 12 ——

A FINAL WORD OR TWO

I have been studying the 8 EV for well over 20 years now. I am well aware that there is more to learn. I don't speak or read Chinese so I only have someone else's translations to learn from and I am supremely fortunate to have had two wonderful teachers, Jeffrey Yuen and David Chan, who supplied me, in English, what I can only describe as life-changing information. To be in the line of transmission from these amazing teachers has altered my understanding of who I am and how I practice.

I have come to really appreciate the archetypal nature of the vessels and I have worked hard over the last 20 years to embody these vessels and cultivate the virtues of these vessels in my life. I believe that you can only give as good as you've got. You can understand the theoretical nature of the Ren Mai by reading the books on the subject. Until you have conceived of something, given your life's blood to gestating it, labored long and hard to bring it into the world and then let go of it in a way that it can live its own life, you may not really "know" the Ren Mai. You can understand the implications of individuation and separation as they are reflected in the Du Mai but until you have been brave enough to face your fears, pull yourself upright and walk towards those fears with courage and will, you have yet to embody the Du Mai. I encourage you to embrace the nature of these vessels in your life. I encourage you to meditate on them. I encourage you to cultivate them by any means. Treat yourself to 8 EV treatments. Take your destiny into your own hands and read some of the books on the 8 EV that teach you Qi gong practices that open and cultivate the 8 EV. Learn how to use essential oils, sound or color to open them in yourself. They are well worth any amount of effort you make to gain a deeper understanding of them.

These vessels are elegant, powerful and ultimately deeply rooted in your curriculum. Embrace them and your destiny unfolds. As a Gemini and a Fire Monkey these vessels have brought me something I never expected. I spent my earlier years plagued by boredom, always looking for that next interesting thing to study or to engage. These vessels have brought me the gift of knowing I will never be bored again. Life is a wonderful adventure. Living in a body is a fascinating although sometimes uncomfortable experience. Emotions and pain are powerful teachers and I try to listen to them with a little more grace and a lot more acceptance than I ever expected I was capable of experiencing. The 8 EV have given me a context for understanding my life, my journey, in a way that always leaves me with the knowledge that I am indeed perfect just the way I am and that I can spend the rest of my life building a deeper and more loving relationship with myself and the world around me.

Could I have done this without the 8 EV? Of course, but as an acupuncturist, they have provided a wonderful and elegant way of understanding the desire for spirit to be earthbound in a body. They are a lovely way of describing how we struggle to be human and how spirit drives us to share our light in the world.

I hope you will be inspired to embrace them wholeheartedly and I truly hope that these vessels will speak to you in a way that helps you to help your patients. I hope you will have an opportunity to experience and understand the profound therapeutic space that can be created by these vessels. You are a light in the world. You have chosen a vocation that attempts to ease the suffering of others and embraces their humanity. I hope these vessels support you in embracing your own humanity and the divinity that is your authentic nature.

Now, someone call the midwife. I think I just gave birth.

Oh wait, there is an 8 EV for that. Never mind the midwife, I think I'll call my acupuncturist.

SUGGESTED READING LIST

Ann Cecil-Sterman (2012) *Advanced Acupuncture: A Clinical Manual*. Classical Wellness Press.

Giovanni Maciocia (2006) *The Channels of Acupuncture*. Churchill Livingstone.

Claude Larre, Élisabeth Rochat de la Vallée (1997) *The Eight Extraordinary Meridians*. Monkey Press.

Dr. David Twicken (2013) *Eight Extraordinary Vessels, Qi Jing Ba Mai*. Singing Dragon.

Elisa Rossi (2007) *Shen: Psycho-Emotional Aspects of Chinese Medicine*. Churchill Livingstone.

Gabor Mate, MD (2010) *In the Realm of Hungry Ghosts*. North Atlantic Books.

Caroline Myss (2003) *Sacred Contracts: Awakening Your Divine Potential*. Three Rivers Press.

INDEX

Page numbers in *italics* refer to figures.